TURNING
TRAGEDY
INTO TRIUMPH

METAHABILITATION: A CONTEMPORARY MODEL OF REHABILITATION

BY JOYCE MIKAL-FLYNN, ED.D., RN, FNP, MSN

Cover design by: Marc Cruz
reachme@justlookdown.com

Front and back cover photography by:
Michael Halfhill of Journey To Awaken Photography
www.journeytoawaken.net

Back of book formal picture by:
Gino Creglia of Gino Creglia Photography
gino@photosbyg.com

Writing and editing assistance: Erin Ryan

Book interior design and layout: Vanessa Perez
books@vanessaperezdesign.com

For information contact: www.MetaHab.com or jmikalflynn@comcast.net

Library of Congress Cataloging-in-Publication Data
    Turning Tragedy Into Triumph
        MetaHabilitation; A New Model of Rehabilitation/Joyce Mikal-Flynn
Includes biological references and index.
ISBN: 978-0-98550062-7
1. Rehabilitation 2.Therapy   3. Philosophy

Care has been taken to confirm the accuracy of information presented. Each person's story was confirmed prior to the publishing of this book. Utilization of their stories was approved by each verbally or in written confirmation. Some information was adopted from their own publications as referenced in their story.

TURNING **TRAGEDY** INTO **TRIUMPH**

For the physicians who kept me alive, the many, many friends who held me up during recovery, my parents, Jude and Mary Joyce, who taught me resilience, and my courageous family, Terry, Elizabeth, Catherine and Keenan, who truly brought me back to life.

You are my heroes. I love you all.

INVICTUS

Out of the night that covers me,
   Black as the Pit from pole to pole,
I thank whatever gods may be
  For my unconquerable soul.
In the fell clutch of circumstance
       I have not winced nor cried aloud.
  Under the bludgeonings of chance
    My head is bloody, but unbowed.
  Beyond this place of wrath and tears
   Looms but the Horror of the shade,
And yet the menace of the years
  Finds and shall find me unafraid.
It matters not how strait the gate,
  How charged with punishments the scroll,
I am the master of my fate:
     I am the captain of my soul.

—W. E. Henley

TABLE OF CONTENTS

CHAPTER ONE

CHAPTER TWO:

CHAPTER THREE:

CHAPTER FOUR:

CHAPTER FIVE:

CHAPTER SIX:

TURNING **TRAGEDY** INTO **TRIUMPH**

PREFACE

Sitting in front of Picasso's Cubist masterpiece, *Musical Instruments and Fruit Bowl on a Pedestal,* I thought of Scott. I wondered if he has ever seen it, the crush of objects broken down and apart, abstracted and reassembled into forms we know but struggle to recognize. Without being forced to examine every angle, every color and texture, I doubt he would know how to put them back together in a way that makes sense. I doubt anyone would.

Scott is a friend and former teammate of my son Keenan. They played soccer in college, and both dealt with injuries that put them on the bench. Scott's knee forced him to sit out the entire fall season of his senior year. He got over that. He came through the disappointment. His knee healed, but the following spring he suffered two concussions on the field. Then, during a boat outing that summer, he hit a wave hard and suffered a third. Doctors gave him advice about soccer—basically, don't play. Concussions have an additive effect, and though no one knows the full extent of these injuries or how they might impact Scott in the future, there is a definite risk. If he suffered another there could be long-term neurological consequences.

This was not supposed to happen. As Scott told me, he knew at some point it would be over, but he always thought he would make that call. He would choose to quit playing because he was tired of it, or because he couldn't get on a team; or a coach would simply tell him he was no longer good enough. Instead, he was forced to make the devastating, very personal decision to stop playing a game he has loved from childhood and planned to pursue professionally. He never thought he would need a backup plan.

Neither do those who survive the most severe physical and emotional traumas or even come back from death. Major or minor, the unexpected strikes. Those in its wake have information to gather and choices to make. Their caregivers, from clinicians to loved ones, must be mindful that they are collaborators in this process. We can provide data, advice and recommendations, but we must be aware that crisis shakes the very core of an individual. If you have never been a 22-year-old soccer player with career-ending injuries, you may still sympathize with Scott, but he is the only one who knows the scope of his loss, the degree to which his life was irreparably thrown off course. Whatever the gravity of the trauma, time must be taken to digest, grieve and process.

At the beginning of this journey there is fear, anger, sadness, confusion and disbelief. I know because I experienced all of these things after my own brush with death and shockingly difficult return to life. It is my goal to help those going through crises focus instead on the gift of MetaHabilitation ©, the process of building new lives that transcend what is left behind. As in Picasso's painting, the deconstruction is what allows, over time, reconstruction in any way they choose. Things may look different, but the essential pieces are there.

This book provides a way, a system for organizing thoughts and behaviors around the notion of overcoming catastrophic events or personal crises and achieving positive outcomes and growth not in spite of them, but as a direct result. During my own recovery and research I was inspired by brilliant psychotherapists Viktor Frankl, Abraham Maslow and Carl Rogers, real-life heroes Abraham Lincoln, John McCain, and Christopher Reeve, and the tenacious survivors who will tell their stories in the pages to come. With unwavering determination, unbelievable stamina, eternal optimism and sheer guts, they transformed terrible circumstances into strength and deep appreciation for life. Tragedy into triumph.

ASSUMPTIONS

Over many years of contemplation and dedicated research since my accident, I have developed six assumptions to elaborate on and clarify the concepts behind MetaHabilitation. They are adapted from Tom Greening's 1964 work on "The Five Basic Postulates of Humanistic Psychology."

1. Major traumas, personal life crises and catastrophic events all disrupt an individual's status quo. Adjustments of biological homeostasis and self-concept are required in order to effectively address the disequilibrium.

2. Such profound existential experiences provide human beings opportunities for significant physical, intellectual and spiritual growth and development.

3. Human beings possess the ability to adapt and ultimately become stronger when faced with severe disruption or danger to their homeostasis.

4. Human beings have the potential and capacity for this resilience.

5. Evidence of it is found extensively in the evolutionary, biophysical world.

6. Human beings innately are or can become goal-oriented, possessing an awareness of their power to influence events, seek meaning and creatively reconstruct the future.

INTRODUCTION

One of my favorite thoughts attributed to Catholic theologian John Henry Newman is that growth is the only definitive sign of life. As a scientist, I know that growth occurs and life thrives in the face of adversity. When confronted with environmental stresses, for example, populations of healthy organisms change and adapt. The populations get stronger (Franz, 2002). To meet the challenges of time, life must constantly reach.

Trauma and disease disrupt an organism's equilibrium, ushering in a chain reaction of behaviors needed for survival and adaptation. This requires not only an adjustment of biological status quo but also an adjustment of selfconcept so that the disequilibrium can be addressed. Rehabilitation, as a modern biomedical model, views trauma and disease primarily as malfunctions of life. Such a view doesn't consider how these events operate as unique, subjective and potentially transformative life experiences.

In an effort to combat this lack of understanding, to promote the notion of personal life crisis as positive and transformational and to adjust the current concept of rehabilitation, I have developed the concept of MetaHabilitation. It identifies and explains the process of individuals who move beyond basic survival and recovery to multidimensional development. Over time, they find meaning in suffering, recognizing the purpose of trauma and, ultimately, the upside.

Prior to a traumatic life event, an individual's level of selfknowledge and selfawareness can cause him to underestimate his own potential. This is why, so often, survivors initially struggle through dependency on others and the disempowerment it engenders. It is at this time that they must face fears and limitations both presumed and real. It is a chance for them to learn who they are and, more importantly, who they can be.

But the concept that devastation and disempowerment can lead to selfactualization is not well known or accepted, and it is underutilized in traditional medicine and rehabilitation. Attention tends to focus solely on pathology, though as Abraham Maslow (1976) asserted: "Man has a higher and transcendent nature, and this is part of his essence, i.e., his biological nature as a member of a species which has evolved." To overlook or deny the very real possibility of such an event prompting a significant growth experience is more than shortsighted. It can hinder a survivor from getting back to productive life.

That is why research was and is still needed in this area, to discover why and how these events drive transformation. Patient care, as well as current health and rehabilitative services, can benefit from the study of personal behaviors and the identification of factors and conditions that improve a survivor's capacity for enhanced recovery. This book explores and analyzes the experiences of six such survivors, with the goal of revealing how they accomplished MetaHabilitation. Human beings have always had the capacity for it, but there has never been a guide for clinicians, survivors and the general public to treating traumatic events as growth opportunities, collaborating with others in achieving recovery, and fostering a mindset that there is no limit to possibility. The only limits are due to fear and frustration, feeling alone and unique in your struggle. In sharing the stories of MetaHabilitated survivors, I hope to instill optimism in those who are struggling, those caring for them and those supporting them. Through profound challenge, all may discover profound meaning.

CHAPTER 1

LIFE AFTER DEATH:
MY STORY

On July 20, 1990, my heart stopped beating. And for 22 minutes, I was dead.

We were at a championship swim meet. My husband Terry and I had been in the stands with 2-year-old Keenan, cheering on his sisters Elizabeth, 8, and Catherine, 7. It was a two-day event, and the second day involved a fun relay for parents. I gathered a team and insisted on swimming the last leg. After all, I told my teammates, I was the fastest.

There was a burst of applause as I touched the wall. Then something happened. I sank, 13 feet down to the bottom of the pool. At first, no one noticed there was a problem. Then it became clear. I was not surfacing. Immediately, Terry was in the water, locking his arms around me and swimming me to the surface where, just moments before, I won the race.

A physician named Stuart Gherini had been racing in the lane next to mine, and he helped pull my body onto the pool deck. He determined that I was not breathing. No pulse. He called for help as he began CPR, pumping blood through my vessels and keeping my brain alive. Fortunately, a handful of other parents were physicians, including an emergency room doctor named Bruce Gordon and an

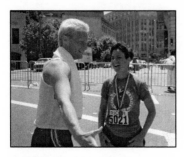

First Marathon with friend, Kurt — San Francisco Marathon

orthopedic surgeon named Garrett Ryle. As my husband and children watched, the doctors took turns and regained a very weak pulse after 22 minutes. A rescue helicopter landed in the football field next to the pool and sped me toward the nearest trauma center. My family and friends watched it take off, not sure they would see me alive again.

I have no recollection of any of these events. I do not remember being in the emergency room or the ICU. My first memory occurred after being transferred from the ICU, out of the trauma hospital to a telemetry floor in another hospital. I was completely unaware of the date or time of day. I woke up to the faces of Jerry and Susan, my brother and sister-in-law.

"Where am I?" I asked. I had no idea what happened or where I was, and it was a question I would ask repeatedly without remembering the answer or that I had asked before. They politely told me, "You had an accident and are in the hospital. Do you want anything?" Strangely, I recall feeling famished and longing for one of my favorite meals, a cheeseburger, French fries and vanilla shake. Although I knew what I wanted, it did not come out that way. I actually remember visualizing it in my head, but I could not say it. I gestured and tried to find the words. "I want, you know, those things that you put stuff on, you layer things on it like yellow and red stuff, and it goes with long things that you put salt on and a cup of that cold, white stuff and you can drive through places to get them," I said. Thankfully they were patient and able to figure it all out. Little did I know at the time, but this was to be my life for a long while.

I was 35, an avid marathon runner and triathlete with no personal or family history of cardiac or respiratory problems. Yet here I was, having suffered something I shouldn't have suffered. That I survived was just as mystifying.

The tests were numerous and painful, but neither they nor second, third and fourth opinions could tell me why this happened. I was left without much information or hope of returning to the life I once knew as an athlete and a professional, as a wife and mother. No one could tell me the exact nature or cause of the cardiac arrest or predict, with any certainty, what my future would hold. They weren't even sure if I had a future.

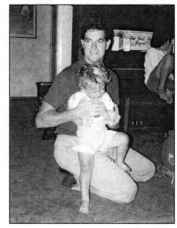

Keenan and Terry — Trying to keep it together with "mom" in the hospital

Although extremely grateful to have been brought back, I found my return to life profoundly challenging. The doctors who resuscitated me worried they had left my family with someone who would never regain consciousness or would be completely incapacitated. While I escaped those fates, I battled cognitive delays, severe depression, physical limitations, intense anger, spiritual angst and consuming fear. Memory loss kept me in a fog. Initially, I didn't recognize my husband or my children. Lifelong friends came to visit, and I struggled to remember their faces and never remembered their names. I did occupational therapy before returning home from the hospital but got frustrated and angry when I couldn't perform simple tasks. Even heating water in a microwave was suddenly, vexingly impossible. This tripped anxiety and overwhelming fear. I understood just enough to know that I was in serious trouble.

I sat with the cardiologist in charge of my care while in the hospital to talk about my future. I asked him about running again, to which he simply replied: "You will never run again. You can walk, but you will never run again." When he left the room I broke down in tears. *This cannot be happening.* He left me with no hope. What was going to happen to me? Later that evening, I saw him in the hallway. I walked up to him defiantly, stating, "You don't know me. I have gone through many bad things in my life and come through them all. I will come through this. You don't know who you are talking to!" I turned abruptly to walk back to my room but could not find it. I heard him say, "Wow, she is yelling at me and she cannot even find her room." I sounded tough, but really I was overwhelmed by fear that he might be right.

I experienced limitations, both perceived and real, that spun me into a very deep depression. I couldn't participate in the athletic events I had enjoyed so much in the past due to very real fatigue, lack of medical clearance and anxiety about the odds of what happened once happening again. To have one of the greatest points

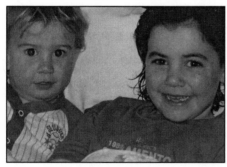

Keenan and Catherine

of pleasure and pride in my life taken away from me and constantly dread that any overstepping could result in another cardiac arrest was overpowering. The life I knew dissolved.

My hospital stay lasted almost a month, and when I got home I didn't recognize it. Standing in front of my closet I had to ask my young daughters, "What outfits and shoes did I like to wear?" In the kitchen, I would look around and ask, "Where did I keep the dishes and the silverware?

What meals did I prepare?" I was lost in my own home and completely exhausted. Friends came over to help care for my children because I literally couldn't. Neighbors took turns bringing dinner. That was wonderful. I did not have the energy or memory to cook.

I spent most of my days sleeping, and when I did find energy to go out for a walk I got lost in my own neighborhood. After a week of this, I decided I was not going to let it get the best of me. I was going to run again. The first time

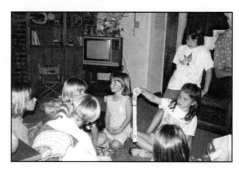

Elizabeth's birthday party, while I was in the hospital

I went I made it two blocks. I had to sit on the curb and recover before I could even limp back home. I was filled with panic, which turned into anger. In the past, I was the one in control and keeping things going, and now I could barely do a fraction of what I had done before. Unsure of what this meant for them, my husband and young children tried to help out and move forward. But all of us were shaken.

A speech therapist came to help me with aphasia, a loss of ability to clearly articulate and understand the spoken and written word. Angry and frustrated, I blamed her for my lack of abilities and refused to continue. With every attempt to resume normal life, I was made more aware of the limitations preventing it. I made a series of poor decisions—something I would later learn is common in people who have suffered brain trauma. I was caught speeding with my children in the car, a reckless act that was way out of character. My husband saw the ticket and said, "Something is wrong with you. I am not sure what it is, but we need some help."

I went to a therapist to deal with my deepening panic and to get some answers about my behavior. I shared with him that since my cardiac arrest occurred in a very public place, I would be out and about and people would stop me and ask, "Aren't you the woman who had the accident at the pool?" Or they would point at me, saying, "There is that woman who had the accident." It was unnerving. It was as if I was some sort of celebrity.

"You are," he said, "but it came with a huge price tag, didn't it."

Luckily, Dr. Daniel Van Hamersveld became my cardiologist and friend. He is a runner and understood my need to be active. He sent me to cardiac rehabilitation. Although I was the youngest by many years, I became close to the other patients. We were all trying to return to life. The intensely monitored activity allowed me to begin exercising, knowing I would not die. That was important. Later, Dr. Van Hamersveld sent me to another cardiologist, Dr. Roger

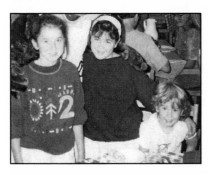

Elizabeth, Catherine, and Keenan one year after my accident

Winkle, who specialized in electrical problems of the heart to see if we could get a clear diagnosis and find out what exactly happened that day. This doctor spent a long time reviewing all of my tests, prior examinations and hospital records. He asked about my life prior to the accident and listened to me. He looked intently at me and simply said, "I have two things to say to you. First, you are the luckiest person I have ever met. I have never met anyone who had that much CPR and is alive and sitting up speaking with me. Secondly, I am afraid we will never really know what happened to you, but your life has changed forever. Your life will never be the same. But it is your life and you can choose how to live it." He reviewed strategies regarding care and post recovery lifestyles. He truly collaborated with me taking into consideration my life and desires. I was frustrated that he did not have an exact diagnosis, but giving me permission to make decisions about my life

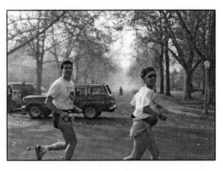

Terry and Me running in the California International Marathon, 17 months after my accident

changed everything. I felt like I had some control.

I was always fiercely independent and strong. I had come through other troubles and challenges. But this was bigger than anything. I met my match. Now, with some sense of control, I realized that the energy I had needed to be focused on some kind of future. It was time to shake off my ego and resentment and move forward. A second speech therapist came at my request. I began to work in earnest, because now I understood the impact of the brain damage I had suffered when my heart stopped doing what it had always done.

I was physically exhausted much of the time, pissed off and completely angry with God. I was almost entirely dependent on others to make decisions for me. My children and husband had to guide me through daily routines. But nighttime was the worst. *You died, and no one is sure what happened* replayed over and over in my head. *What if it happens again?* I was in constant fear of death.

Six months after my accident, this feeling of impending doom washed over me. I could not take it. Although I was still angry with God and had not sincerely prayed since my accident, I gave up. I had to. I had no other choice. I got out of bed and down on my knees and pleaded. *God, take these feelings away from me. I cannot*

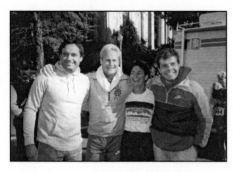

California International Marathon before my accident, with Mike Crosby, Kurt Carpenter, and Jim Wohlleb

live with this fear anymore. I got back into bed and slept peacefully through the rest of the night. That fear, that sense of doom, has never returned to that degree since that night.

After about three months, I felt ready to return to work as a nurse practitioner. But my first day back I got confused on my way to the office. I worked on a very limited basis and was disorganized and slow in making even the simplest diagnosis. I had to constantly review all of my cases with colleagues. They were extremely patient and always made certain things were done correctly. Although I desperately needed help due to cognitive delays and fatigue, I was given no information or guidance from within the medical community about what to expect. I was alone.

I remember driving home from work one night, about nine months into recovery, feeling very tired, frustrated and scared that I would never regain what I had lost. Staring at the darkness on either side of the road, I let it creep into my thoughts. *I just can't go on living like this. I don't want to go on living like this. If I just drove my car into this embankment, it would all be over.* But I didn't. In that moment, what stopped me was an overwhelming thought, a realization that I could not do this to the people who had worked so hard to get me back—all the medical professionals and therapists, family and friends. They had sacrificed and given so much just to give me a chance. I couldn't do it to them.

The loss of cognitive and physical ability, memory and control in all areas of my life was overwhelming and frightening, not only for me but also for my family. Not being fully aware or informed of the ramifications of such loss was almost worse. Thankfully, with the passing of time, intense determination, speech and occupational therapy, cardiac rehabilitation, my own creative rehabilitative interventions and counseling, I was able to return to much of the life and activities I had known before everything went black. I began to accept the accident and all that came with it, reflecting on, reinterpreting and eventually developing an appreciation for what once seemed like the worst thing that would ever happen to me.

Slowly, I found my way back into the world. I participated fully in my children's school, sports and social activities, gaining a profound appreciation for everyday pleasures. I successfully resumed my work as a nurse practitioner but now felt I needed to do more. So I pursued a master's program in nursing to challenge myself and to formally investigate the survivor's journey.

While I was inquiring at Sacramento State University, the chair of the Department of Nursing, Dr. Robyn Nelson, happened to come into the reception area. It was a fluke. She heard me tell the receptionist about my reservations, as I had been in an accident that caused some brain damage a year earlier. I had significantly improved, but entering an advanced degree program was not going to be easy. Dr. Nelson stopped and asked my name. As soon as she heard it, she froze.

"Are you the woman who drowned at the swim championships last July?" she asked.

"Yes," I answered.

"I was there," she said. She took me into her office. We talked about that day, my life now and what I was hoping to do. Eighteen months later I earned a master's degree in nursing, completing a thesis: *A Phenomenological Investigation of Near Death Event Sur-*

vivors. Dr. Nelson was an adviser on the project and later served as a consultant on my doctoral dissertation committee. Our paths intersected again when she hired me as an assistant professor. My event brought us together in many ways. She has become a loving friend and trusted mentor.

Before my death and slow rebirth, I judged myself only on what I had accomplished—how fast I could run or how much I could fit into a day, spending little or no time enjoying. While I had established good relationships, I had failed to prioritize what was essential for a healthy life. I never said no to anyone's demands or requests. I always tried to add more hours to the day. This way of living left me exhausted and frustrated and, I believe in a major way, brought about my accident. I always looked at what I was missing, focusing on my shortcomings and failures. I didn't see the forest through the trees.

Now I see both, and in a completely different light. I consider every day a gift. I rarely get through one without stopping to appreciate the fact that I am alive and able to share my life with family and friends. I focus on what I can do. I listen to advice from doctors but temper it with my own desires and awareness of my abilities. I was given back my life—a very meaningful, purposeful and fulfilling life—something I had been told not to expect.

I recently reached my 50th birthday. While out for a run, I thought about it. *Wow, 50 years old.* Then the insight came to me that rather than bemoan my age, I should celebrate it. I was elated that I was able to *be* 50. I remembered a quote from the book *Miracle in the Andes* by Nando Parrado (2006). It's about a young rugby team's plane crash in the mountains on their way to a game in Chile. The survivors were stranded on a glacier for months before two of them braved 45 miles of frozen wilderness to get help, including

Nando. His father, thinking the whole time that his son had been killed, met him at the hospital and said, "The sun will come up tomorrow and the day after that and the day after that. Don't let this be the most important thing that ever happens to you. Look forward. You will have a future. You will have a life." I made the choice to define my life by how I lived after the accident. That was what was important, to celebrate and create *my own* future.

Despite my impressive recovery, I was unsettled. From clinical and personal points of view, I felt strongly that the information and interventions offered to me were insufficient in facilitating a complete physical recovery and addressing the event itself as a unique opportunity for emotional and spiritual growth. I had experienced this growth and recognized it many times in patients I cared for, as well as in books and films. The survivors had in common a belief that such events could give more than they took away. What prompted this unique human behavior? What was involved in this power of the human spirit?

Driven to answer these questions, I embarked on another academic journey 10 years after earning my master's. It entailed further investigation and a formal study of why and how these critical life events can and do prompt significant growth and development. I wanted to understand exactly what this power is and how it works. I thought it might open the door to a new way of thinking about and using catastrophic experiences by revealing how they bring forth a deeper appreciation of self and life. What is this spark inside us, I wanted to know, and how do we tap into it?

So I entered a doctoral program with the unambiguous intent to investigate what I call enhanced survivorship. I was assigned an adviser, a professor to help direct my studies and guide my research. But due to shifting teaching opportunities, I was assigned a new adviser on three different occasions. I ended up changing course, too, pursuing research on post-cardiac events and rehabilitation. It was worthwhile, but it was not what I had entered the program to do.

I met with Dr. Dean Elias, my third and, thankfully, last adviser, to discuss my project. I presented him with more than 100 pages of work I had completed and was prepared to research post-cardiac care. We talked for a long while, going over the specifics of what needed to be done. Just before leaving the meeting and quite by accident, I said, almost as an afterthought: "Here is a paper I wrote for a research class. It's an idea I have about rehabilitation; it's called MetaHabilitation, a word and concept I've been working on. It has to do with the belief that when a person is faced with or challenged by a catastrophic or deleterious life event, he has the capacity to actually grow and become stronger as a direct result of the event." He knew my background and took the paper. One week later, we met again to firm up the details of my cardiac research. He looked directly at me and said, "You know, this cardiac work is interesting, but this MetaHabilitation concept is amazing. This is what you need to do." I was not happy about the prospect of starting over. Nonetheless, I took some time and thought about it. He was right. This was my passion. This was where everything was rooted.

After much exploration, collaboration, consultation and deliberation, the concept and model of MetaHabilitation crystallized in my dissertation, *Transforming Life Crisis: Stories of MetaHabilitation After Life Crisis*, which is the foundation of this book. My family threw me a lovely party to acknowledge its completion. Many friends were there, including a few of the doctors who kept me alive on that July day.

Bruce Gordon was among them. I had run into him many years before, shortly after the accident. At the time I said, "You know, Bruce, I think I have brain damage." He smiled and said in his reassuring way, "Joyce, I have never resuscitated anyone who actually walked up to me and said, 'I have brain damage.' All those neurons in your brain are still there, they are just not firing fast enough. You are an athlete. Just like when you have to rehab a sports injury, you have to rehab your brain." As soon as he said it I understood, and I worked diligently to do just that.

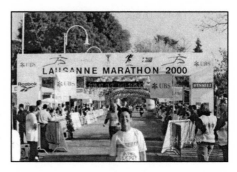
Me running the Lausanne Marathon, 2000

At my doctoral celebration, after I publicly thanked people and briefly discussed my research, Bruce walked up behind me and whispered, "You know that brain damage you had? I think it's gone!" He smiled, and I knew the journey had been completely worth it.

My life is full. I have seen all three of my children graduate from college, all Division 1 athletes, two in soccer and one in water polo. I watched both daughters walk down the aisle and have been blessed with grandchildren. My son, who was a baby when I almost left him forever, is a man. My husband Terry and I celebrated over 30 years of marriage. I continue to teach; interestingly enough, one of my courses is in neuroscience. I never gave up hope. I talk about that with patients. I never take their hope away. It is the fuel that allows us to survive and motivates. Don't take that away. They, as I did, will figure it all out.

I continue to run and have completed several marathons, including California International Marathon, Venice, Lausanne and ran along with friends in the Boston Marathon. I have finished three triathlons. While I participated in these events, it was not with the same intensity or level of competition as in the past. And it didn't matter. I am alive. The joy comes not from how fast I run but from the running, the doing. I learned a new way of thinking about and understanding life and earned a deep appreciation for the power of the human spirit—of my spirit.

These are the gifts I was given.

CHAPTER 2

METAHABILITATION:
A CONTEMPORARY MODEL OF REHABILITATION

M odern medicine is powerful. Due to sophisticated and constantly evolving technology and pharmacology, there is an optimistic outlook for survival from many significant diseases, traumas and even catastrophic life events. Nevertheless, after the initial recovery, anxiety and emotional distress set in, requiring survivors to continually adjust. They and their supporters must recognize and reconcile the impact of the event and adapt to the uncertainties of a future that may bring chronic physical and psychosocial problems. Trauma and crisis are inescapable aspects of existence. Some are more brutal than others. The human ability to take a positive stand against adversity introduces dimensions of consciousness that allow for redefining and reinterpreting the meaning of these growth experiences (Frick, 1987).

The current rehabilitation model tends to view such adversity as a malfunction of health. But that health is defined solely as "useful" activity, negating a person's ability to face, overcome and make meaning out of malfunction. Failure to derive meaning creates, as Viktor Frankl (1992) wrote, "an existential despair and spiritual distress rather than an emotional disease or mental illness. This, however, in no way implies that we must discard and abolish the medical model. What we must do is simply recognize its limits."

Through my own experience as a survivor, I recognized these limits. I lived them. And I came to understand the benefits of my accident, the potential for selftransformation, selfactualization and personal mastery. As nursing theorist Margaret Newman noted, "disruption in human beings, such as disease or catastrophic life events, often become catalysts, potentiating the unfolding of life processes that persons naturally seek, thereby facilitating movement from one pattern of consciousness to another and transformation into order at a higher level or expanded consciousness" (Newman, 1997). Not only was the disruption key to my transformation, the desire to make sense of it was a totally natural one, even when it involved depression and anger. Had these insights been presented as part of the recovery process from the beginning, they could have made a major difference in the amount of time I spent despairing as opposed to digging in my heels and moving forward.

The idea of enhanced recovery had been with me for quite some time, but the exact concept came into focus quite suddenly and accidentally. I was reviewing an X-ray series of a fractured tibia, showing the initial break and several stages of the healing process. In each film, I saw reflections of myself.

Even though a bone is strong, it may fracture or break if subjected to excessive weight, sudden impact or stresses from an unusual direction. Most fractures heal, even after severe damage, provided that the blood supply and the cellular components of the bone survive. After a fracture, whether partial or complete, extensive bleeding occurs and a hematoma develops. Next, an internal and external mechanism produces cells that stabilize the bone. These cells are replaced by new bone. Fragmented ends are united.

With appropriate therapy and time, this region will naturally be remodeled and little evidence of the fracture will remain. The recovery may continue, almost unnoticed, for up to a year. If the initial injury is allowed to heal properly, the site of the fracture becomes stronger than the surrounding bone (Fredrick, 1998). Years later, X-rays will reveal that a fracture occurred, but if supported correctly the repair of the bone is complete. In that one spot, it becomes virtually unbreakable.

This phenomenon is present throughout the biophysical world. Even bacteria mutate into stronger strains in order to survive. Whole ecosystems reflect this capacity. As I began to further contemplate and understand this process, I saw it everywhere. I noted such transformations and enhanced healing in all areas of my practice and life. Some of the patients I cared for and others I read about experienced healing not just for the purpose of survival, but also to ward off intrusions to their homeostasis or health. My colleagues engaged with me in long clinical and intellectual discussions to clarify the concept, and MetaHabilitation took shape. *Meta* is a Greek word that denotes going beyond. *Habilitate* refers to ability, with rehabilitation meaning to restore. MetaHabilitation recognizes that people can surpass or exceed simple restoration following an existential phenomenon.

However, the phenomenon is not the focus. The MetaHabilitation model acknowledges the severity of a traumatic event, with its unimaginable spectrum of physical, psychological and spiritual pain, but ultimately promotes the survivor's mastery over that pain and gratitude for the resulting insights and enhanced inner strength. The event is a moment of before and after, a pivotal point. MetaHabilitation uses that point, building on the inborn human capacity to endure and find meaning in the worst.

THE PROBLEM

Humanistic clinical psychologist Clark Moustakas (1977) believes that at the base of every person is a candle that lights the way, burning with all of our energy and power. He also believes that when life takes a devastating turn, *we* are the ones who either stoke or snuff out our own flames. Some survivors never get over being negative and bitter about what they've lost. Others manage or even strive to move beyond the negative, and a few become personally enhanced or enlightened. How do we explain these very different outcomes? What is it that enables one person to improve his condition, to move beyond basic survival to find meaning and purpose in the trauma and life afterward—to MetaHabilitate?

Survivors have done it in all eras of human history. It is not really a new concept, yet there is a notable lack of information about and attention given to this form of recovery in the current model of rehabilitation and health care in general. Also lacking is research focusing specifically on strong, welladjusted patients and on comprehensive health rather than pathology. There is limited inquiry as to why some people choose to view these life events as transformative, and we know even less about how they transform.

The purpose of my investigation was to discover the why and how of MetaHabilitation. My method was to dissect the exact experiences of survivors—as seen through their eyes—and the recoveries that led them to a higher level of functioning across the spectrum. I hope this information will make a contribution to the fields of rehabilitation and behavioral medicine. It is essential to generate new, more progressive ideas and interventions to expand treatment options and promote a more complete picture of recovery. My goal is to reduce the burden for survivors by providing a system that allows for the normalization of this process by framing major life events and subsequent healing as a meaningful, transformational experience.

STAGES OF METAHABILITATION

In attempting to answer the question of how one MetaHabilitates, I was constantly amazed by how gracefully and courageously my subjects moved through the stages. That doesn't mean there were no challenges, problems, depression or times when they simply did not want to go on. But they recognized these times and ultimately chose to overcome rather than succumb. What is even more striking is the fact that these people did not simply recover. They went far beyond. An actual metamorphosis occurred. Having no conscious choice in the problem and yet courageously navigating the solution is remarkable. It is a lesson for us all.

Through interpretation of the data I collected, six stages of MetaHabilitation emerged. Stage one is acute recovery. This involves the immediate and emergent aspects of care necessary for survival. Once survival is ensured, questions about expectations for the future begin. They are tough and difficult to answer, and though survivors struggle, they eventually come to a turning point—the second stage. They say yes to life and consciously choose to move forward. They actively participate in traditional rehabilitation programs provided at this time. Stage three involves ongoing therapeutic interventions. Once the choice has been made to live and move forward, the survivors and families are very involved in seeking out treatment modalities both complementary (nontraditional) and traditional. They look at whatever might bring a cure or resolution or reduce the burden of the event. Acceptance and adaptation encompass stage four. Once therapies have been utilized, survivors acknowledge, at least for now, what they have left. Once they accept, they adapt to the situation and are willing, able and eager to return to life. In the fifth stage they go back to the life they knew, to some extent, depending on their capabilities. They strive to return at the highest level possible and focus on living a happy, productive and useful life. It is after some time that full recovery happens, the last stage of taking on the future. Survivors have moved forward, accepted and now embrace the event. The journey of recovery has given them so much insight into their own strengths. They recognize the support and love that allowed them to heal. Appreciation for all of it and an enhanced understanding of what life is about occurs in this final stage. They are MetaHabilitated.

The decision and determination to transform their lives and future are not automatic. Therefore, answering the question of why MetaHabilitation occurs is required as well. To begin, most of the survivors I interviewed had backgrounds of hardiness and resiliency. What they did not absorb in childhood they achieved later in life. Unbelievable positive outlooks moved them toward MetaHabilitation. Failure to respond to challenges blocked the path to a new life. They threw off obvious or invisible ties and let go. They also soaked up tremendous support, advocacy and love from those around them. Particularly strong at the beginning of their recovery but also during other points in time, friends, family, doctors, nurses, coaches and support groups, even dreamed visits from deceased relatives, carried them. Positive books, movies and prayers helped them believe that they could and would move on and become stronger. They left no stone unturned. They forged on despite limitations, looking at progress, not exactness.

In the following chapters, you will meet some of the people who truly inspire me. Their stories serve to illustrate each stage of MetaHabilitation, with updates on their lives today revealed in the epilogue. Whether you are a survivor, a loved one, a health care provider or just a curious soul, I hope you'll begin to appreciate what they paid such a premium to understand.

CHAPTER 3

STAGE ONE
SURVIVAL: ACUTE RECOVERY

On a Saturday morning, Jerry flew to Mexico with his 15-year-old son Michael. They checked into the Galapagos Inn, a dedicated dive resort. Scuba was Jerry's passion, and though his wife Gail and daughter Jamie were also certified divers, this was a special trip just for father and son.

On the fourth day the conditions were perfect. They dove with a group, 100 feet under the warm, jewel-green waves for 18 minutes on a computerized clock. Jerry started the ascent with the dive master, making the appropriate stops at different depths to "gas off." Because of the intense pressure underwater, the gases inside their bodies were compressed. Nitrogen had dissolved into their blood, and if they rose too quickly, bubbles could form, expand and stick inside their vessels. But they did everything by the book. Fifteen feet below the boat they made one last stop to take care of any lingering gases. They got the signal to rise, but before Jerry reached the surface his right arm went stone dead. Given his training as an endodontist, or root canal specialist, he thought he was having a stroke. Michael had to help him onboard. A few minutes later his breath sounds were so weak that a certified EMT on the boat was ready to start CPR, but after several minutes of oxygen therapy Jerry recovered.

Hooked up to a steady stream of oxygen, Jerry was able to raise his right hand by the time the boat reached the shore and a waiting ambulance transported him to the local hospital. His Mexican caregivers did neurological tests for eye and hand coordination, and everything seemed normal. They decided to observe him until they could be sure he was out of danger. After a few hours of rest, they asked Jerry to walk forward and backward. He was a little unsteady going back, and his doctor recommended time in a decompression chamber, where his body would be taken back to dive pressure so any residual bubbles of nitrogen could gradually shrink and dissipate. He walked into the chamber unassisted at 5 p.m., still wearing his bathing suit and flip-flops. Nearly six hours later, the techs told him he could come out.

"I was like a dishrag. I could not move. My legs were paralyzed, and I had to be pulled out of the chamber and lifted onto a gurney," Jerry recalled.

Now he was scared. He told Michael to track down two American trauma doctors they'd met at the hotel and were supposed to dive with the next day. Michael brought them to the hospital, where they proceeded to evaluate Jerry's condition. They administered what is called a pin test. Using a safety pin, they started at Jerry's feet and moved slowly up both leg and sides of his torso. They reached his chest before he felt any sensation. At that point, the Mexican doctor who originally examined him came into the room and told Jerry he would be fine in the morning.

"You are not fine," one of the American doctors said when they were alone again. "You are in real trouble. You have T-4 spinal cord damage."

When morning came, Jerry's new friends literally stole him out of his hospital bed and rushed him and Michael to the airport, where they'd commissioned a medical jet with the help of the Diver Alert Network. After bribing the Federales to let them onto the tarmac, Jerry and Michael were bound for Houston.

An ambulance was waiting when they landed to rush them to a specialized hospital in Galveston that cares for people with spinal cord damage. Jerry spent a month there, with his family by his side. He was totally paralyzed from the chest down and spent time each day in the hyperbaric chambers used to treat the decompression sickness suffered by Galveston's large population of oilrig workers. He had fairly good use of his hands, except for a constant tingling in the fingers on the right side, but the damage to his spinal cord had caused irreparable damage to his legs. The first "hit" he took, Jerry told me, was likely an embolism—a blockage caused by a tiny bubble of gas. When it passed, probably on the way to the Mexican hospital, his body became functional again. But something happened after that, while he was in the decompression chamber. And he'll never really know what.

He was left with no feeling in and no power over his legs, not to mention his bodily functions. He spent most of his time in Texas learning to use a wheelchair, a catheter and suppositories, and how to manage the constant, tingling fire in his extremities. He did another six weeks of intensive rehab at a hospital near his home in Sacramento before getting down to the business of what the rest of his life might look like.

The first time he left his house after that was for a Halloween party, where many of his friends would see him in a wheelchair for the first time.

"I spent the evening seeing everyone at belly-button level. That was the level that I was at, for the first time in my life, not standing," he said. "You have a different view of the world when you're in a wheelchair."

But Jerry still believed he could come back from the paralysis, and he threw himself into physical therapy twice a week. He learned to balance on the parallel bars, and he remembered staring down, blown away by the fact that his feet, which had moved him all over the world for more than 50 years, could not even be lifted to take one step.

MetaHabilitation and basic rehabilitation begin with acute medical intervention. This is a very intense time focused on basic survival, and it is laden with emotions and tough decisions for the survivor and his family.

Once survival is assured, they begin the process of dealing with the aftermath. What is gone? What do they have left? What challenges lie ahead? There is distress, fear, disbelief and confusion. For the survivor, there is a sense of having little to no control over his condition and life. He will undoubtedly ask himself, why me? Unfortunately, there are no good answers in this initial stage.

Jerry had been a successful, fit, middle-aged dentist with his own practice. That person died on the beautiful morning of August 26, 1992. Now he was an incontinent, impotent, depressed survivor stuck in a wheelchair. As he told me, there are support groups for people suffering from heart conditions or drug addiction. There is nothing for the handful of people who get in accidents while scuba diving. Not having someone to talk to who really understands can make a person feel utterly alone, even surrounded by those who love him.

Stuck in a new and unwelcome reality, that loneliness can turn to hopelessness. Over 30 years, Jerry had defined his life—and himself—by his career. Every day he rose at 4:30 a.m. on the dot, with routines scheduled into exact, repeating increments: Gym, coffee, shower, work, home, repeat.

"That's the way I functioned, and I loved it. And I still miss it," he said. "That part of my life was in control. Then I had no control."

Without full function in his hands, Jerry was finished as a dental specialist. Pouring all of his energy into recovery, he tried to engage in old hobbies, but he could no longer focus well enough to read or play the piano or listen to good music. As the months went by and he felt no closer to escaping the prison of his own body, he found himself wishing for release—the same kind I had wished for driving along that dark road.

"I realized I was depressed, unbelievably depressed. One day when I was alone in my house I thought, *I don't want to go on anymore; I don't want to live any more, this is crap.* I have a .38. I took it out—it's a revolver, so it doesn't miss, doesn't get jammed up—and I started playing with it. Then I thought, *this is nuts; you can't do this; you've got a wife and two kids.* I put it down, reached behind my bed, grabbed the phone," Jerry said. He told me that was the lowest day of his life. It was also the day he called a friend about setting him up with a psychologist. "I said I was having a problem and needed to see somebody really badly. I put the gun away but certainly reached a feeling of futility and got to the point where I considered ending it all. For many years, besides my therapist, I could never discuss with anyone what happened that rainy afternoon."

Survivors, especially those who were very self-sufficient before their lives were altered, have trouble recognizing or admitting that they need help. That's why those around them must provide it without even being asked, reminding them that there is a world outside the one that's collapsing. Formal counseling with a therapist able to deal with post-traumatic grief is essential. This therapy focuses exclusively on moving forward. It acknowledges that something significant happened and then closes the door in order to open others.

Jerry started seeing a therapist after he made that first call for help, and he continued seeing one every week for a long time. He availed himself of medications that helped with hypertension and erectile dysfunction while simultaneously exploring alternative treatments, from acupuncture and nutrition to a consultation with a Mexican shaman—something he would have found dubious or even laughable before his accident. He contacted the American Hyperbaric Association, and its librarian sent him everything she had on dive accidents, including the fact that unlike other types of spinal cord injuries the "spotty hits" he suffered were not beyond regeneration.

He also connected with another survivor, one who suffered blindness and paralysis after a similar dive accident. They vented to and supported each other over the course of a year, and even though the other guy made a nearly complete recovery, Jerry knew he understood better than just about anyone what it was like to be inside his head. Despite myriad frustrations and setbacks, Jerry never stopped visualizing his own healing.

"I would lie in bed, close my eyes, fold my hands over my chest and envision the nerves in my spinal cord regenerating. I used to do that at least every day for about 15 minutes, when nobody was home," he said.

Slowly, he cut his visits with the therapist to every other week, then once a month. But it was the personal relationships that kept his spirit alive, the family and friends who believed in him when he was too weary to believe in himself. Survivors must be presented with enormous amounts of love, support, optimism, opportunities, goals and, most importantly, hope. They must be afforded as much control over their situations as possible and encouraged to collaborate and participate in decisions regarding their care. The burden is carried, for a time, by those around them, but only to give them a chance to gain strength in order to take over the task of recovery.

Jerry learned to drive all over again with hand controls. The first time he urinated normally he cried. And he cried even harder in the bathroom of an Italian restaurant, where he was celebrating the birthdays of his wife and son. It was there that for the first time in two years he had a real bowel movement, thanks to trying an alternative medicine nutritional diet. It was right around that time that he learned to walk with canes, even though he still had no feeling in his legs. He remembered one of his doctors, who was also a dear friend and neighbor, coming to see him every single night in the weeks following his accident.

"He kept saying, 'You are going to walk again.' That was an awesome, unbelievably positive statement," Jerry said. "And I did."

CHAPTER 4

STAGE TWO
TURNING POINT: SAYING YES TO LIFE

In the early days of WWII, grenades and bullets were already flying through the windows of David's house, some by the hands of neighbors and former friends. He was the youngest of eight children, a Polish Jew literally caught in the crossfire of a world gone mad. Before the war even started his parents installed a solid mahogany door plated with steel, but nothing could protect them from what was coming.

It took the Nazis less than three days to wipe out the entire Polish Army. David's only brother Abraham, nicknamed Romek, was "one of the lucky ones" taken as a prisoner of war. Although he served time in a concentration camp, he was among a handful of prisoners released on the condition of exile. Instead, Romek joined the underground resistance. The Gestapo repaid the young rebel by torturing him to death in front of David, who was only 13 at the time. They let him live, but only so he could run home and tell his mother what they had done.

The family left everything they owned to hide with David's uncle in the city of Tarnów. At dinner one night, he met a pretty young woman named Helen, who told him when the war was over she hoped to marry his cousin. While they were eating, the door blew off its hinges. The Nazis opened fire with machine guns. Helen landed on top of David, her body shielding him from the bullets.

His aunt and uncle, his cousins and nearly everyone else who lived in the 18-story building were murdered in a matter of minutes. By some blessing, his parents and siblings had been out that afternoon. When they returned and found him huddled in the massacre, there was no time to clean off the blood. They ran.

And they kept running, to an old auditorium, then a vacant warehouse, then an abandoned apartment. His father was eventually caught and killed while doing forced labor for the Nazis. David's mother continued to hide him and five of his six sisters until the morning boots crashed against the door. David slid under the ragged sofa just as the whine of rifle shots filled his ears and the smell of gunpowder overwhelmed every other sense. Booted feet stopped inches from his head. He heard muffled German. Someone laughed. One soldier even jumped on the couch, slamming the springs into David's stomach, but he didn't move or make a sound. He finally turned to look at the bodies on the floor. Aside from his eldest sister Rachel, who had escaped to Europe before the war started, his entire family was gone. In his book, *Because of Romek: A Holocaust Survivor's Memoir* (2005), David wrote about that moment. "I lay down on top of Mama, put my arms beneath her stiff body, and held her close. 'I promise you, Mama, I'll live. I'll survive, and I'll go to London and find Rachel. I'll tell the world what they've done to us. I will Mama, I promise.'"

After wandering for a time in the city, then 15-year-old David found an encampment of rebels in the forest and joined their cause. He ended up falling into the hands of the Gestapo, who sent him to a concentration camp.

"Two men were holding me very tightly. With their nails and some kind of mechanical ink they were digging into my arm, over and over and over again, sometimes close to the bone with that nail, with the letters, 'Auschwitz Concentration Camp ... 161051,'" he remembered.

Inside the transport, more than 100 people were crammed "like herring," standing for almost 20 hours without rest. The train doors finally opened onto the road outside of Auschwitz, where the guards ushered their prisoners in with wooden bats. They had a German shepherd that mercilessly tore into anyone who got too close.

"Before he was murdered, my brother was teaching me. He says, 'David, when you come in front of these Nazis selecting people, remember, you speak well German. Speak up; maybe they let you live,'" David told me. In crisp German, he lied and told the guards he was a 21-year-old metal mechanic ready to work for them. One laughed and then brutally beat the boy with a rubber hose and a cable. Even though he was cowering on the ground, David felt the dog chomp down on his right leg. When a soldier pulled it off, a chunk of David's bloody flesh was hanging from its teeth.

The Nazis took so much more from him. They forced him to prep cans of Zyklon B, the cyanide-based poison used to gas his fellow prisoners in droves. Once they were dead, David was tasked with scouring the bodies for gold, from wedding rings to the fillings in their teeth. One day, an infant child survived and was still suckling at her mother's breast when David pried the woman's fingers apart. He and another prisoner tried to smuggle the baby back to the women's barracks, but they didn't make it far. The other man was killed on the spot. The baby was tossed in an oven, and David was tied to a chair and beaten with hoses and bats. He was ordered to count every blow out loud, and he did so until he could no longer speak.

"They untied me and threw me down on the floor. Colonel Adolph Eichmann, who came to see his progress, with his hands on his hips like this, he looked at me and he said, 'You wish you were dead and your problems will be over, but you're going to die anyway. First I make you sick; I make you suffer.'"

Throughout the Holocaust, David cheated death and the despair that coiled around the hearts of so many others. He had survived nine concentration camps by the time Allied forces freed him from Bergen-Belsen. He was 18 years old and weighed just 72 pounds.

After the war, his sister Rachel sent for him, and he began training as a baker in England. He traveled to France to hone his baking skills, and when he returned to England he landed a job with the House of Commons. The head chef there, who was French, was grilling him about his skills with soufflé. After everything he had been through, he took it in stride. It helped that Winston Churchill was there to back him up.

"He said, 'Have you ever burned anything?' And I said, 'Yes, your honor, more than once.' And he said, 'Chef, why are you wasting time? This is the man you want.'"

David also fought in several wars for Israel. He contracted polio, and the doctors who treated him were sure he would either die or be crippled for the rest of his life, but he beat that, too. He was married more than once and had children of his own. His book about the Holocaust became known throughout the world. It was part of that promise he made to his mother, to survive and never forget.

"Millions of people died. There was so much torture. They could not take it any longer. They gave up. People went to the barbed wires and they committed suicide. They could not take it," David said. "I thought many times to do that. But somehow I said no. I <u>promised</u> my mother. It was like something came over me, something told me not to do it."

Three times he was sent to the gas chamber to die, and each time, the guards turned him away, saying he would get his shower tomorrow. Outwardly, he looked like everyone around him, an emaciated, broken ghost. Inside, his candle flame never stopped burning.

MetaHabilitated survivors can often identify a turning point, a moment of crucial insight that helped them realize they had a choice about what path to take. This is the start of developing a desire to move forward and make plans, to actively work on recovery. They begin to see that the meaning of the trauma transcends everything it inflicted. In this second phase of recovery, they stop asking, why me, and start asking, what now?

Many attribute their strength to their upbringing—the influence of parents and teachers, the bonds of faith, the memories of past adversities that tested their mettle and proved they could endure and overcome. But in this case, and so many others, it was the promise. If you ask David what saw him through so much hatred and unbelievable heartbreak, he'll tell you that he made three promises, one to his brother, one to his mother, and the last to an iconic French rebel named Fania Fénelon, who was forced to play music outside the gas chamber at Auschwitz where David should have perished along with so many millions of others who didn't have the impossible strength, the will that could not be crushed. She said, "little boy, I have seen you three times and three times you have been sent back. Promise me you will survive".

He made a choice. He promised them that he would live, and he kept that promise.

CHAPTER 5

STAGE THREE
TREATMENTS: CONVENTIONAL
AND COMPLEMENTARY

Connie was no stranger to sickness. In 1978, when she was only 32, she battled breast cancer and lost her breast. She spent almost 20 years as a social worker, working with individuals struggling and living with developmental and mental disabilities. And her husband John succumbed to multiple sclerosis, leaving her to raise their two children on her own.

The disease turned his body's immune cells against his own nervous system. Inflammation ate away at the protective sheaths around his nerve cells, and the signals that controlled everything from balance to bladder function slowed and eventually stopped. It was a gradual, horrible way to die. Connie was powerless to stop it, just as she was powerless to foresee the event that almost took her life in the blink of an eye.

John's family was rooted in Croatia, and after he died she wanted their son Matt to see it as their daughter Stacey had years before. It was the summer of 2004, and two weeks into the trip they decided to make a detour to the island of Hvar. They rented scooters to tour its coastline, and though she rode for hours, Connie kept saying that something in her vehicle's mechanics didn't feel right.

Rounding the corner, almost back to the rental place, she felt the scooter's engine rev out of control. The power surge sent her flying off the road, over a cliff.

Connie's helmet came off in the air, and she landed 40 feet down, on her head. Unconscious but alive, she had a split skull; most of her teeth were missing; her right eye was blown; and her jaw, hand, arms and ribs were broken. She was covered in blood and splinters of her own bones. Matt was the first to reach her side. With the help of family, some bystanders, and a makeshift stretcher they carried her body up to the top of the mountain.

A helicopter was called and arrived almost immediately. On that particular day for some unknown reason, the crew included a doctor who instantly intubated her. While the emergency responders suggested they drop Connie at the local hospital, the doctor knew that her only chance of survival was to reach the big trauma center in Split. Because of the Yugoslav Wars fought in Croatia in the 1990s, the staff there was trained for high-caliber trauma. A helicopter delivered Connie into their hands.

Matt and Stacey were by her side when she woke up from the coma. She has virtually no memory of the 10 days she spent in that hospital or the long trip back to California to complete her care and recovery. But with crystal clarity, she recalls the conversations she had with her dead husband John, who was also in the room, even though he had been gone for almost a decade. In fact, the day she was discharged was the 9th anniversary of his last day on Earth.

"I remember being with John during that time. I don't remember being in the hospital; I don't remember the circumstances. I just remember being together and being happy and walking and talking and being warm in the sun," she says. While they walked through the space between, John told Connie how proud he was of their kids and that it wouldn't be fair for her to leave them without a parent. That message went deep, tapping into the spirit that had always defined her. Stacey saw it shining through, even as her mother lay motionless and unconscious. Years later, she expressed the marvel of it in this letter:

What can I say about my Mama and her recovery that would enlighten or inspire? I almost feel as if I needn't say a word. That she is more powerful than words. But since she was there, I will tell you this; the woman I saw in the hospital was physically, spiritually unrecognizable. I don't think I have ever seen anyone hurt so badly in my life, and it was my Mama, my inspiration, my support, the person I love most on this planet. She was struggling to say the least. As we sat with her and watched her and talked to her, beneath all the pain, trauma, wounds and vein injuries, so was the essence, the essence of this wonderful joyous, loving, brilliant woman that shone through. In these moments, no reasonable human being would have even tried to convince us that she was going to be okay. I knew she would. That kind of radiance cannot be extinguished. My mother is powerful beyond her own comprehension or recognition. She will say it was us who brought her back, and that may be true, but only because she sacrificed for us knowing that we need more time to walk in her light. Shine on, my sweet Mama, you are a star. I love you beyond words.

As her husband John reminded her in the dream, she had to come back. And she did. Powerful though she was, Connie went through a phase of complete dependence on those around her. She couldn't drive for eight months. She could barely walk. This was a woman who had climbed Mt. Kilimanjaro and Mt. Whitney, Machu Picchu and the Grand Canyon. She was a runner and avid softball and tennis player. And her life had been devoted to serving those less capable. Now she couldn't get around her own house.

"I have always been like a walking encyclopedia of names, numbers, everything. When I first came home I had sticky notes everywhere. I had to remember to eat; I had to remember to feed the dog; I had to remember to do things that, for the most part, you took very much for granted," she told me. "I didn't even know who I was for a while. So people really surrounded me with lots of help and lots of positive energy and lots of strength."

But asking for help was extremely difficult. She had spent her whole life helping others, always being the rock. Her independence stemmed from the fact that she was adopted when she was just two weeks old. While her adoptive parents were kind and loving, she says, "There was always a sort of missing piece." It drove her to develop an inner strength, one that both hindered and helped her recovery. At first, she had trouble accepting help. But she came to understand how vital it is.

"To learn to ask for help was very big," she said. "I was very fortunate to be surrounded by people that were very happy to be givers, and I was able to be a receiver."

Once the turning point occurs, that choice made to live and move forward, survivors and their families get very involved in seeking treatment—whatever might bring resolution or just reduce the burden. Often, this takes the form of traditional medical treatments and rehabilitation of physical functions and behaviors. It moves you back into life by helping you learn about yourself and your abilities. As time passed and her energy improved, as with Jerry, a continued push to find any and all pathways to recovery - traditional and complementary took precedence. Being open does not mean being foolish. Consultations were a part of the process and making informed decisions was essential. But there was an enthusiastic drive to explore options for recovery and healing. It gives the survivor a sense of control and hope, both essential.

Connie had "dark days," but they were outnumbered by "sunny days" that reminded her how much she wanted to stick around and enjoy life with her loved ones. Just as she had going through cancer and her husband's long illness, she naturally focused on the positive. She did physical therapy 2-3 times a week for almost a year and yoga a couple times a week. She sought out formal counseling. She faithfully hit the gym. She challenged herself and seized more and more control over her life, reintegrating in whatever ways she could. Some things she learned from therapists, some she was exposed to through interactions with kindred survivors, and some developed through basic trial and error. She listened and took advice but only if it supported her efforts in meaningful recovery. It was a very courageous and productive time, but there was room for grieving. She understood how important it is to reaching the next stage of life, and not just for survivors.

In this stage of MetaHabilitation, thoughts have serious weight- they become actions. "Thoughts become things. Think good ones. Choose good ones," Connie says. "I do think it is important to go through a grief process, and I think part of that is you get sad, you get angry, you get confused. I think it is important to acknowledge that and to deal with that and to sit with that and then try to move beyond that. ... Don't think about the things you don't have but focus on the things that you do have. My life is different, no other way about it. It is different. So I said, 'Okay, this is the life that I get now, and it's good.'"

She understood her crisis affected others close to her. "It was as hard on the kids as it was for me, I think, to talk about it, to process it, to put it out there, to go through it. Not relive it, relive it, relive it, but be able to talk about it. I think you go sort of piece-by-piece, or hurdle-by-hurdle, or rock-by-rock. You get up the path," Connie says. "Physically, I probably did die. But I think much of me came back. … I think my essence is still here, and a big part of that is due to Matt and Stacey being there and being with me to help me come back to where I was."

CHAPTER 6

STAGE FOUR
ACCEPTANCE AND ADAPTATION:
A TIME TO REFLECT

He was always the shortest one on the team. But Dominic was strong and feisty as well, thanks to being lovingly brutalized by his two older brothers and to the inspiration of his parents, who immigrated to the U.S. and built a successful business from nothing.

"I definitely have a passion for the underdog," he told me. "I have always been friends with people that are optimistic and think that they can do anything.'"

That's why Dominic believed he could get into the University of California, Berkeley—even though he didn't have the grades—and start for its powerhouse rugby team—even though he didn't have the size. His academic progress after a few months at a junior college was enough for Berkeley's dean of admissions, and his strength, speed and sheer nerve on the field impressed the rugby coaches. At 22, he was living his dream.

That Christmas, Dominic was still on top of the world. He felt invincible. And after a night of drinking with friends, he decided to get in his car and drive the mile or so back to his house. It was 2 a.m. and a storm was ripping through, but he figured it was worth the short drive to spend the night in his own bed. So he hopped in the old family Suburban. He remembers looking down at the speedometer, which read 35 mph. That's when the Suburban spun out, the force building and building until a massive tree stopped it like a sledgehammer.

"I knew instantly," Dominic said. "I was paralyzed."

The road was empty, and the rain was so loud that even the car horn could barely cut through it. Dominic honked and screamed for about 15 minutes before a figure appeared in his window. He woke up in the hospital. He still couldn't feel his legs.

"I remember asking a nurse if I would ever walk again, and she didn't say no but she didn't say yes," he recalled. He would come to learn that with spinal cord injuries, that answer is standard. Even for specialists, it's impossible to know what kind of recovery will be made, especially right after trauma. Dominic chose to feel hopeful, imagining he would be one of those patients who would make an odds-defying return to full feeling and motor function. But his spine was 75 percent separated. Surgeons had to fuse it back together and align it with steel rods on both sides. After a month of recovery and rehab in the hospital, he realized that the time had come where he should be getting ready for spring rugby. Many of his teammates visited. Their words were encouraging, but there was something in their eyes, a kind of sadness.

Despite the difficulty Dominic was having in rehab, he was still convinced the final outcome of his ordeal wouldn't be that bad, that his life would go pretty much back to normal. Then his doctor told him his paralysis was not temporary. He went over Dominic's options, what he could and could no longer do. He didn't tell him that he would never walk again, but there was little comfort in the prognosis. Dominic said it was like a bad dream. And from what he could tell, he was never going to wake up.

His family took him to a center in Vallejo that focused on re-habbing spinal cord injuries. Unlike the hospital in Sacramento, where he spent most of his time in bed, this place was all about preparing him for his new life in the real world. He relearned how to get dressed and get in and out of a car, which was strangely comforting considering what had happened the last time he was behind the wheel. It made him feel like no matter what, he could be independent again.

He was there for more than a month, his mom and sister bring-ing food every day and his dad and brothers dropping by almost as often. His teammates drove down all the time, and while he ap-preciated the attention, he finally asked them to stop.

"It's hard to not be normal … you don't necessarily want to have people see you vulnerable. You don't want people to see you when you are struggling," he said. "I needed to figure things out for myself before I could share my struggles with people besides my family."

Figuring things out involved a lot of Internet searches for infor-mation on alternative treatments. Dominic's mom found something called laser puncture that was happening in a little French town called La Charte, and many testimonials swore by its effectiveness. It wasn't until they left California that they realized how accessible the state is for the disabled. Dominic was hit between the eyes with all the challenges he would face if his paralysis didn't improve.

"I remember when I was going to France, being on the plane and trying to deal with everything, and I just remember thinking, instead of looking at the obstacles that might come up, I would try and take it as a journey," he said. "I didn't know what the hell I was going to do and how I was going to live with this and all that, get-ting away from seeing my friends go along with their daily lives and my family doing what they always do, and going into a different environment on a sunflower farm in the middle of nowhere. My closest neighbor was miles away. There was a lot of time to think, a lot of time to read and just clear my head and figure out some things. ... I would see people that are paralyzed from the neck down and little kids that couldn't move their hands, and they were still happy and were still living life. That was inspiring to me, being able to think about things, get away from all the chaos that kind of surrounded my accident at home."

He travelled back and forth to France for about a year, undergoing treatments that were essentially acupuncture applied with laser technology. Another patient hadn't moved her fingers for 30 years, and he was there when she wiggled them for the first time. Even though he desperately hoped for this kind of result, being with so many other survivors helped him appreciate what he had. While he regained some feeling in his lower back and hips, he said the therapy turned out to be much more powerful mentally than physically.

"I remember in France thinking about, if this could happen to me, if something this bad could happen to me, why couldn't something great happen to me? ... For every bad thing there is something good that could happen, too."

The first good thing was Dominic's decision to move to San Diego. He spent a lot of time on the beach and made great friends, coming to a new kind of normal. He didn't leave his old life completely behind, but it was important for him to feel like he had the time and space to redefine himself, without anyone who knew how much he'd lost feeling sorry. Even though it's a natural response to pity a friend or loved one after a trauma, it's the worst thing for that person to see the doubt they already feel on every face that comes in the room.

Dominic became even more active than he had been before his accident. He biked and learned to paraglide, went skydiving and swimming. Even though the lower half of his body didn't work, the rest of him was strong, and his resolve to live a good life was stronger. Beyond his own journey, he began thinking about what he could do to help others in his situation feel so empowered.

Acceptance and adaptation—these are the keystones of stage four of MetaHabilitation. Once therapies have been utilized, survivors acknowledge, at least for now, what they are left with and what they must deal with on an ongoing basis. They get back to life.

Dominic was lucky to have an innately optimistic disposition and a family that supported his recovery. But the key for him, in stark contrast to Connie, was removing himself from the familiar. Life goes on, as they say, and he needed to stop in order to face the truth. He went to a place that fit his needs and engaged in activities that facilitated growth and meaningful participation in life, not as a disabled person, but as a fully functioning individual.

"I remember my coach coming into the hospital room when I was in Sacramento, and we were talking about college, and he asked me if I was going to finish up and this and that. I had no clue at that point. I was thinking probably not. I remember him saying, 'You've got to go back.' He's a big six-foot-seven rugby guy, and he said, 'You've got to go back into the lion's den.' That actually always stuck with me," Dominic said.

Even though staying in San Diego and enrolling in college there would have been easy and fun, Dominic returned to Berkeley. He finished his degree in American Studies, with an emphasis on business and entrepreneurship. That gave him great confidence, but some of the most crucial aspects of his recovery came from dedicating himself to helping others with similar disabilities, especially other rugby players with spinal cord injuries. He founded the Try For Others Organization, which provides financial assistance to buy equipment ranging from custom vans to workout equipment and wheelchairs. The idea, Dominic told me, is to help people with physical challenges recognize they can be active again, to "get their blood flowing and let them enjoy life a little bit more."

To raise money for Try For Others, Dominic did a 45-day bike ride from Florida to San Diego, supported by two able-bodied riders, including his brother. His father drove along with them. His family and friends stopped noticing the wheelchair, and Dominic ultimately realized that its limitations were largely up to him.

"I have been put in so many situations where people kind of expected me to feel this way or expected me to feel that way and were always trying to tell me what was good for me, when I knew for myself. A lot of times there were doctors and physical therapists, and they were trying to tell me, you need to this or you need to that, you need to take this or take that. A lot of the times they were correct, but other times I had this strong feeling that they were just completely full of it, and I always regretted if I didn't go with my gut and I didn't trust myself," he said. "I truly believe I will walk someday. … If you have any hope, it's not false hope."

CHAPTER 7

STAGE FIVE
REINTEGRATION: RETURNING TO LIFE

Y ou have breast cancer. A sentence no woman wants to hear. But Suzy heard it, and at a young age. She was 35, a wife and the mother of three young daughters. How could this happen?

When she found the lump a few months earlier, she wasn't too concerned. She worked for a surgeon, and when the appointment she made to have it checked got bumped for an emergency procedure, she didn't even bother to reschedule. She got busy and distracted and just forgot. Lucky for her, an errant golf ball literally knocked some sense into her.

She had met her husband Joe in Arizona. He was there for business and golf, and she was there to soak up the sun. After a few hours by the pool, she went up to their hotel room and found a note. Joe had written that if she went out on the balcony and looked through the trees she might catch a glimpse of him teeing off. As she stood watching, a golf ball came out of nowhere and hit her so hard in the forehead that it knocked her into a wall. Her immediate thought was that she'd been shot. Bloody and panicked, she called down to the front desk for help and ended up at the local hospital for stitches. Mysteriously, the ball was never found, and no one on the golf course recalled losing one that day.

Suzy asked the surgeon she worked for to remove the sutures about a week later. While she had his time and attention, she casually asked if he might also evaluate the lump in her breast. He sent her for a mammogram immediately, then a biopsy. It was cancer, another form of the disease that had taken her father just a year before.

"I know my father threw that golf ball from heaven," she says.

During her lumpectomy, Suzy experienced another stroke of luck. Her doctor happened to do a blind biopsy and found a second tumor even closer to her chest wall. It was much more aggressive. Left unchecked, it could have meant the difference in her very survival. Because of the size of the tumors and the associated risks, the doctor recommended a double mastectomy. The cancer hadn't yet spread to her lymph nodes, so Suzy was able to spend the rest of the summer with her kids before going through the surgery and six months of chemo. As she had been about their grandfather's disease and death, she was very straightforward with her daughters about what she was going through. Although she had moments of profound fear, she wasn't angry or disillusioned. She assured her kids she was not going to die.

"I don't think I ever did the 'why me?' I just didn't go there," she said.

It helped that she had a friend to confide in, someone around the same age who was diagnosed at the same time. They even had the same doctors and, as Suzy says, "walked the same path together." But her friend's cancer spread to her femur. She was dead within 18 months. The loss hit Suzy hard, but she was determined not to let depression consume her. After having both breasts removed, she remembers being agitated and sick from the anesthesia. Her family stepped out of the recovery room, and she had some time to sit and just breathe. Suddenly, the room lit up and warmth washed over her. She says she was not alone, that God was there, telling her she was going to make it. Her resolve to surround herself with positive things, people and thoughts grew even stronger.

"I did not watch sad news; I didn't read sad books. Everyone was sending me funny cards to make me laugh, which was so helpful. It was amazing to me what people did for us, the little, thoughtful things," she said. "I think it's important not to isolate yourself, to be around as much family and friends as possible, as long as they are not negative and as long as everybody has good energy, positive feelings. … If you have any spirituality at all, reach out for that and surround yourself with good thoughts and good laughter and as much positivity as possible."

When her father was diagnosed, Suzy started looking deeper into prayer and contemplating heaven. She had never been one to talk to God on a daily basis, but she found herself doing just that. She also joined a prayer group that was a source of great comfort and support during her own battle with cancer. One of the books they read interpreted the Psalms, and Suzy connected with metaphors about a maple tree in winter drying up and losing all of its leaves in order to come back again in the spring, and sheep that couldn't drink from a stream until their shepherd had "damned" the water. She figured her water had been damned so she could drink, and she found herself extremely nourished by what her struggle did to strengthen her faith and her gratitude for every moment and tiny pleasure.

When she started chemo, the nausea was overwhelming. Despite the enormous amounts of help she was getting from Joe and her friends, Suzy was so sick that she felt her children would be neglected. This devastated her more than any of her own suffering, so she asked for help.

"God says commit and trust Him, and He will bring it to pass. … We don't even think about when we mail a letter; we just take it to the post office and put the letter in a mailbox. You just assume it's going to get there. We trust that it is going to get there," she told me. "I spent the entire Saturday in prayer, just saying, *I am giving this to you. I can't be sick and have three little kids. I can't do this. So, there it is. Help me out.* That night I had a dream about an uncle who recently died. He was a physician and said to me, you need to take your anti-nausea medicine every morning before you even lift your head off that pillow. He was giving me this advice, and I woke up the next morning and said to Joe to get that medicine. From then on, I took it every morning and never got sick again."

Suzy's body responded well to the treatment, and a few months after her surgery she had her breasts reconstructed. She has been in remission for 15 years, though she knows that any moment the cancer could return. The thought of dying has never stopped her from living.

"I think that life is short. I do not take things as seriously as I used to. … When you go through something like this it just makes you realize how important everyone is, how important love is, and we may not be here tomorrow."

Given time to grieve, choose a path, start the rehabilitation process, adapt, adjust, reflect and begin to understand what a trauma has meant, survivors move back into life. They choose to reintegrate in a significant way. Their energy is restored and they are physically, mentally, emotionally and psychologically ready for the challenges ahead. To the best of their ability, and always seeking improvement, they go back to school, jobs, families and society.

Even if their lives look much the same as they did prior to the event, they tend to see things differently after this phase of MetaHabilitation. If the crisis and trauma brought about limitations, they reconstruct their lives to fit more comfortably into what they are able to do and move forward. It isn't that they're immune to fear and uncertainty about the future. They simply rise above.

"When I look back at that time of my life I truly feel blessed for the opportunity of that time. ... It was a very quiet, peaceful, restful time in my life," said Suzy, acknowledging that crisis can be a very powerful motivator to slow down, reassess and smell the roses among the thorns.

CHAPTER 8

STAGE SIX
METAHABILITATION:
TAKING ON THE FUTURE

"My mother's story would be, 'Kurt, Joanne, I'm going to have one drink after work and then I'll be home to fix dinner.' Then it was, 'I'm going to have one more drink and then I'll be home to fix dinner.' And then it was, 'Well, I'm not coming home, so take a TV dinner out of the freezer.' From that point, we knew we could do whatever we wanted," Kurt said.

He was just a kid, but the alcoholism both his mother and father suffered from had already infected him. They divorced when Kurt was 7, and his mother's next relationship was rocky. By the time he was in junior high he was drinking heavily, and when he was 17, his older brother gave him his ID, and his mother vouched for it so they could go out drinking together.

"I think having that feeling of less than, what I found in the alcohol was that it makes us feel different, it makes us feel better, it makes us look better," he remembers. "I would do anything or say anything to make you like me, and alcohol, without a doubt, filled that void that I had in my life."

But the void was too big even for alcohol to fill, so Kurt got into drugs. And all of it seemed cool until the night he watched police handcuff his mom and take her to jail for drunk driving. That moment changed her life, but it would take many more years for the seed her recovery planted to bloom inside her son.

The next year, 1975, Kurt moved to Los Angeles to pursue acting. Convinced he was going to be "the next Dustin Hoffman," he craved the recognition he got onstage almost as much as the pot he was smoking and selling. Under the bright lights, he could be somebody else. He was always looking for happiness outside of himself, and that often meant spiraling deeper into his addictions.

In 1979, he was cast in a big role, and he decided to get serious and only get high after rehearsals. At that point, his mother was five years sober, and the thought burned in his head as he drove home from work with a friend one night, both of them stoned. He said he didn't think he could ever quit, that something needed to happen. And, as if by magic, something did.

"I started getting this feeling of what I call adrenaline running through my body. ... This white light came out of the sky and through the windshield, and it hit me right in the chest. I couldn't talk. I was just in awe of what I was experiencing ... I looked at Mark and said, 'You are not going to believe this, but I'm never going to get high again,'" Kurt said. "That was the last time I smoked."

It took him almost 10 more years to give up alcohol. He had married a woman with similar vices, and he started going to Alcoholics Anonymous as a way to get out of the house at first. But he thought of his father, who died from alcohol abuse when Kurt was only 22. And he remembered what AA did for his mother, who became a different person after only six months in the program. Many of the testimonies he heard were about positive things that came from sobriety, from going back to school to reuniting with family. It helped him believe that he could change, too—back into the person he was trying to escape inside the bottle. Because that person had a chance to be better and have a better life. At the age of 33, he gave up his demon.

He enrolled in college, but in order to fully commit to his education, there was something Kurt had to know. He talked to his counselor and asked to be tested for a learning disability. It was the first time he admitted to anyone that he believed he was stupid. That belief was rooted in his being held back from fifth grade.

"What that did to me—it made me feel stupid, made me feel less than," he recalled. "I went literally from being the teacher's pet to the class clown. I just didn't care." And because of his parents' alcoholism, they weren't really present to guide him through the struggle. The cycle of apathy, anxiety and addiction snowballed from there.

Kurt took some tests on a Saturday, and 10 days later the administering psychologist called him in to go over the results. He was terrified that his worst fear would finally be confirmed.

"She said, 'Kurt, you are a smart man.' It was the first time in 40 years anybody ever told me I was smart," he said. "What I realized is I had no self-esteem. I was bankrupt in that department."

The validation made him dream of a life that was bigger than the void he'd been filling with substances, and it also helped him realize that his real problem was not in a bottle or a pipe or a pill. It was inside of himself. After he got clean, Kurt remarried and found rewarding work. He talked with his mom about how feelings of inadequacy had affected his life. She said she wished things had been different for him and that she had made different choices. He told her he wouldn't change a thing.

"I have a life today beyond my wildest dreams. For a kid growing up knowing he was never, ever going to amount to anything,

I have respect today. I have a son who, to this day, has never seen me drink, has never seen me drunk, has never seen me hung over, has never seen me mean or ugly. He has a father today who participates in his life, and that's all I wanted as a kid growing up. I have people in my life today that care about me for who I am and not about the outside stuff. I have a relationship with my mother, with my sister, with my family members. I am so blessed. Today, my cup is half full. My cup is half full all of the time because I have this life that I never ever knew existed for me. I owe it to sobriety. I owe it to the fellowship of Alcoholics Anonymous. I owe it to God," he says. "I wouldn't change anything."

When accomplishing this final stage of MetaHabilitation, survivors rarely return to the beginning, but they occasionally shift back to an earlier stage, mostly as they face new challenges. However, each new success builds on the one before, and they gain more confidence in themselves and their ability to move forward. They go back to the lives they knew, to some extent. They strive to return at the highest level possible and focus on living a happy, productive and useful life. It is after some time that full recovery happens. This is when survivors go beyond accepting the event to embracing it. They realize how much it and the ensuing recovery provided insights into their own strengths. They recognize the support and love that allowed them to heal.

They fail to see their limitations, focusing only on what they can do. They have given themselves time to contemplate the entire event and the recovery process—many times. This is a very philosophical stage prompted and promoted by support from family, friends, therapists, spirituality and religion, personal accomplishments and an ongoing sense of hope leading to gratitude. They see the event as a journey. They have figured much of it out. They have attempted things and succeeded. This success creates confidence, ongoing hope and optimism. They focus on the positive aspects of their lives and what they have to look forward to. They realize that these events did not take away from their lives, but opened up time and space to enjoy and appreciate the things they probably would not have. They have a passion for life and embrace new challenges. They know what is vital. They see the big picture—relationships, spirituality and joy in just being here. They have not only recovered, they are stronger and better. They do not linger in negative thoughts, they let go of the desire for the life they had before and embrace the one they have. They are MetaHabilitated.

CHAPTER 9

THE METAHABILITATED SURVIVOR

Why did these individuals MetaHabilitate? Simply stated, they said yes to possibility. This is critical. They realized there *was* a future, and that led to hope that built on the support of family, friends and health care professionals. It was the holding onto hope, even in a fragile state, that ultimately gave meaning to their lives and allowed transcendence of their critical events. Hope led to different thinking. They developed an attitude, a conviction about the future—they were free to choose. There is a distinction between potential and actuality. We all have potential, but it is recognizing and embracing personal freedom that makes MetaHabilitation more than just a fancy word. Viktor Frankl put it this way: "At the beginning of human history, man lost some of the basic animal instincts in which an animal's behavior is imbedded and by which it is secured. Such security, like Paradise, is closed to man forever; man has to make choices."

These real-life examples prove that almost everything can be taken away from a person, but as long as he can still choose his attitude, there is hope that he can come back from the brink. That point in time when we choose a way, the turning point, rests on an unwillingness to accept the alternative. It is a bit of an enigma to try and ascertain specifically why some choose to move forward and others do not. Perhaps it is lack of support or guidance, overwhelming feelings of hopelessness and despair, or maybe they simply do not have a mindset that was formed, from an early age, to look at things in a positive way. Nonetheless, choices were continuously made. They were choices that helped these individuals move forward constructively, prompted by a sense of necessity, urgency and, at times, fear. They stumbled and suffered disappointments, but they never truly gave up.

Sometimes the conviction was dependent upon the survivor's own strength. Other times, certainly in the acute stage, it came from others. With each success came hope and more control, willingness and desire to push forward. This led to eventual mastery of the situation and allowed for personal contemplation and recognition of where they had come from, what they had and an eventual sense of appreciation for the event. They got it. The trauma gave so much more than it took. It allowed for an opening up of the mind and soul to the truth of what was really necessary and precious in life.

It is absolutely necessary to normalize this process and journey for the survivor. Recovery is not an illness or deviant condition; it is a rehabilitation concern or set of concerns, bringing with it the necessity to reorganize as well as the opportunity to actively recreate the self. During my own situation, Dr. Roger Winkle, stated so clearly and succinctly: "This event has changed your life forever. Your life will never be the same and there are decisions to make regarding how to live that life. But they are your decisions."

But he was in the minority when it came to how my team of doctors treated my condition. What was emphasized most was what I could no longer do or expect to do. The focus appeared to be on lowering my expectations for reentry into the world by stating what limitations I should expect after survival of such an event. The promotion of this negative thought process, and the absence of a positive perspective, diminishes a survivor's capacity to reflect and ultimately reinterpret the experience.

In addition to the lack of understanding and effort on the part of the mainstream medical community and their narrow approach to recovery, there are multiple problems within the health care system that significantly affect the appropriate utilization of current rehabilitation programs. Obstacles to services occur due to lack of regular referrals, payment structures for rehabilitative services and a lack of appreciation and understanding by health care professionals of how important these services are to patients and how these events can provide them a unique existential vehicle.

Years after telling me that I would never run again, and enduring my rebuke in the hospital hallway, my original cardiologist acknowledged the validity of what I said—he really did not know who he was dealing with. A lot of people have told me they couldn't have done what I did. They're sure they wouldn't have the strength. I've been asked countless times: Can anyone MetaHabilitate? And my answer is always an emphatic yes. At this point I know of no specific genetic mutation that negates the capacity to experience an enhanced recovery. It is apparent that some individuals struggle more than others due to their particular crisis, background and lack of support or personal desire. Such obstacles are direct areas to identify and address during the healing process. More may be needed in terms of counseling or therapeutic care. I do not adhere to the notion that there is only one way to do this. I believe the capacity lies within each of us. How it is discovered and tapped into is unique, but there are some characteristic behaviors and thought processes. Understanding them sheds light on how one accomplishes this kind of recovery, allowing therapists and other health care providers to institute the appropriate therapeutic interventions to successfully accomplish it.

MetaHabilitated survivors live with continual hope and gratitude—hope that they will continue to improve, that they will walk again, run, improve their motor skills, be free of cancer, and that they will continue to learn from life's lessons. They feel their lives, even with imposed disabilities or problems, are worth living. They are eventually grateful, profoundly grateful. They are here; they are alive; they can enjoy life. Perhaps not exactly the way they did in the past, but nonetheless, they are still able to be a meaningful part of others' lives and the world in general. They are better, not bitter.

They made sound and productive personal choices and continually surrounded themselves with positive thinking, messages and people. They did not tolerate negativity. They refused to live with anger and despair. They moved on. They stopped asking, 'why me?' and instead asked, 'why not me?' They chose to define themselves not by the crisis or trauma but how they lived their lives afterward.

They grieved what they lost and focused on what they had left. This was accomplished by taking the time to think through things and to remove themselves from familiar surroundings and people in order to get clarity.

They had lessons to learn. What am I to make of this? How do I go about living? Answers to these questions were not always easy or forthcoming. After initially struggling, most asked for and accepted help. They sought the insight and support of therapists, spiritual guides and various health care professionals, which allowed them to accept, adapt and see things with more clarity and hope. They let people in instead of always thinking they had to go it alone.

They accepted what was and moved on. They noted limitations but did not allow them to stand in the way of moving forward and getting back into life. They realized they could function with limitations and still do very well. Although the limitations were frustrating, they began to look at alternatives and recognized how to overcome obstacles. They needed and wanted to move on. They did things despite fear and selfdoubt and experienced successes that motivated and led to further successes. They recognized that the effort, the willingness to move forward, was as essential as the outcome itself.

They made promises to others and kept them. This gave them tremendous strength while facing enormous odds. To surrender to the situation was, at times, a consideration, but eventually strength of will and belief in the future won out. There were bigger issues at hand, people they had to answer to, people they made promises to, people they needed to come back to who wanted them even with incapacities. They had reasons to come back.

They laughed. There were times when families and friends helped them see the lighter side of it all. They enjoyed humorous cards. They eventually were able to laugh at themselves and even at aspects of the situations in which they found themselves. It was essential and allowed them to normalize their lives.

They took time to figure things out. Many had the occasion to remove themselves from day-to-day routines in order to free up energy to heal. They thought it was essential to take time away from work and contemplate. What is this all about? Where am I to go now? What am I to do? Why me? Who am I? They needed to physically remove themselves from their environments and from people who knew them before everything changed. They were different now, in many ways, and needed to figure it all out without people judging or feeling sorry for them. They needed to get away from the small talk and constant questions about what happened. They had much to ponder. One day their lives were moving in one direction and the next, they had changed completely. They needed time to grieve and regroup. They needed to and could make decisions about how to effectively recreate themselves. They gave themselves permission to do so. The hero's journey is an isolated one at times, and these survivors recognized that.

It is important to note that some survivors interviewed for this study had significant financial wherewithal to assist in the recovery process. They had the ability to take time off work, travel to different countries or vacation homes where they were able to rest, recuperate and spend unlimited time in contemplation and reflection—privileges not afforded to all who are faced with similar life-changing events. But recognizing this aspect of MetaHabilitation—the necessity of time away and time alone in order to contemplate—is more essential than focusing on the specifics of each situation. To discard the importance of such behaviors involved in MetaHabilitation because they are not readily available to all is dangerous and shortsighted. What is most essential is assisting people, no matter what their circumstance, in finding or creating such a place for the purposes of quiet, insightful reflection. We know it's important, so families and caregivers should collaborate and find a way to make it happen for survivors, whatever it looks like.

When considering a healing place, we must not center on what we cannot do or what does not appear possible but instead take lessons from these survivors and look at what can be done. Focusing on the negative is the antithesis of MetaHabilitation and should not be tolerated by those in the health care field. Instead, attention must be placed on what has been discovered as helpful and essential in complete and enhanced recovery and how to accomplish this creatively.

Survivors rarely give themselves pats on the back. They are very modest and selfeffacing, crediting all who surrounded them with love, honesty, support and courage with the fact that they have done so well. There is joy in how they talk about their lives now. Even with obvious limitations, they are sincerely happy. The basis for all this is simply love, and they offer it to physicians, other health professionals, family, friends and people they serve in their careers and volunteer work. They understand human connectedness and choose to focus on what they have in common rather than what separates us. They lost so much—professions, money, opportunities, bodily functions and abilities—yet, what they saw as essential in life was fostering and cherishing their connections and relationships with others. During their journeys, they recognized the tremendous love and support provided by others until they could once again depend on themselves.

Lastly, they gave back and continue to do so. They looked at how they could be of service to others who had endured similar situations. This provided meaning in their lives, giving them a mission and knocking out any self-pity. They had been given so much; they needed to return the favor. All the survivors I interviewed had an intense desire to give, to help, to be part of something generative. Also, they noted the lack of services for people in their situations and decided to help fill in the gaps. It made their recoveries more complete.

CHARACTERISTICS

In observing MetaHabilitated survivors and using their experiences as constructive models of recovery, we must be aware that while these individuals achieved extraordinary things, they are as ordinary as you or I am. They and others with similar outcomes may tend toward certain personality traits or have backgrounds, social circles or financial resources that allow them to deal with trauma in a more straightforward way, but recovery is not exclusive.

It is also important to note that there is some overlap between facilitating conditions and characteristics of the MetaHabilitated survivor. The latter includes the following:

1. Grateful.
2. Hopeful.
3. Resilient.
4. Optimistic.
5. Surround themselves with positive, optimistic people.
6. Adaptable.
7. Refuse to live with anger and despair.
8. Accepting.
9. Grieve losses and life changes but ultimately move on.
10. Stop asking, 'why me?' and instead ask, 'why not me?'
11. Seek and accept help from others.
12. Focus on possibilities (continally search for and are motivated by new opportunities).

13. Keep their promises (use reassurances to others as motivation).
14. Define themselves by their lives post-event rather than by the experience itself.
15. Take time to contemplate past lives and build new ones.
16. Insightful (able to gain wisdom about themselves and their conditions).
17. Recognize and embrace personal choices.
18. Review where they were, where they are now and where they want to go.
19. Make sound and productive personal choices regarding care, goals and life.
20. Give back.

FACILITATING CONDITIONS

With the exception of Kurt, the survivors I interviewed all came from supportive families. But as Kurt's story illustrates, strength can also come from outside sources such as AA. Whatever the makeup of "support groups," they promote and model the way for survivors, advocating for them and assisting their efforts in working through troubling events, especially in the early stages of recovery.

The following conditions are powerful supplements to the characteristics that promote MetaHabilitation:

1. Family support, both initial and ongoing.
2. Advocacy from family and support groups.
3. Positive relationships with family and friends.
4. Spirituality (a sense of a superior power from which to draw strength).
5. Willingness, innate or learned, to accept help.
6. Stay away from negative people and thoughts.
7. Surround themselves with positive people and thoughts.
8. Research conditions to receive the best and most up-to-date care.
9. Go with their guts (make very personal decisions about their care and recovery).
10. Exercise significant control over their care and recovery.
11. Take time to grieve losses and figure things out.
12. Accept their conditions—for now.

13. Adapt to the situation and life.

14. Recognize inner strength.

15. Focus on what they still have and can still do, as well as the choices before them.

16. Set goals, both short and long-term, allowing them to redesign their lives as they choose.

17. Get back into life by taking one important step, and then another.

18. Push limits (overcome fear and apprehension and try new things in an effort to improve).

19. Contact others with similar problems to vent and give and receive encouragement.

20. Give back (deep desire to make a difference).

21. Maintain hope for the future.

22. Recognize the gifts brought forth by the experience.

CHAPTER 10

CLINICAL APPLICATION:
METAHABILITATION AS A TECHNIQUE

Direct utilization of this model requires a review of the stages, characteristics and facilitating conditions. At the onset, it is essential to evaluate the person individually, identifying the specific stage he is in to provide proper guidance and normalize the experience as he is assisted in progression from one stage to the next. The intake interview and assessment of each person should focus on and identify:

• The current stage of MetaHabilitation
• Personal characteristics
• Facilitating conditions

Personal characteristics and facilitating conditions are noted in order to support those present and categorize specific areas of intervention. The intake information must also include a past medical and personal history. Each patient is interviewed and assessed regarding specific features shown to support a positive outcome. The stage of MetaHabilitation is determined by the clinician and, at times, the patient and family. Also, during the intake interview, information is acquired as to the presence or absence of each characteristic and facilitating condition. It is vital to advise families about this information, as they are critical, especially in the early stages, in helping patients through the recovery process. This journey is not one to be taken in isolation by the patient and clinician. Families must be involved as they are a part of the crisis and have a stake in the recovery process.

As stages are identified, it is necessary to inform patients of the specifics of the stage and how progression through each is accomplished. There is no specific timetable associated with any stage, just as there is no cookie-cutter approach to each situation. Patients can progress successfully over the course of several months. Again, this progression will involve unique aspects of the individuals and what they're up against. However, if lack of progress is noted, review and regroup is in order identifying and addressing potential obstacle(s) to once again, move in a positive trajectory.

EPILOGUE:
WHERE ARE THEY NOW?

I am the master of my fate:
I am the captain of my soul.
　　　　　— W. E. Henley

I did not think I could be more impressed with the people I initially interviewed back in 2006, but I am! It meant so much to reconnect with each one and listen to where they are now in their ongoing recoveries and lives. I hope you enjoy reading these updates as much as I enjoyed putting them together.

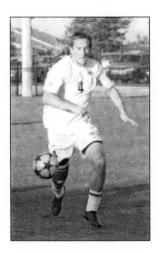

SCOTT

After graduating with honors (cum laude) from Marquette University, Scott became a sales representative for an orthopedic company. His work brought him into the surgical suite. While observing surgeries that utilized his company's products, he was more and more fascinat-

Scott on the field at Marquette University

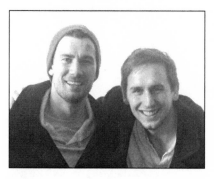

Keenan and Scott at Marquette University

ed and intrigued. This changed the direction of his life. He is currently taking the required courses to apply for medical school. He will complete these prerequisites by 2013 and hopes to begin medical school in 2014. Who knows what discoveries he might make about the injury that ended his dream of playing professional soccer? Despite that, he continues to be active, playing basketball, tennis and golf and training for triathlon. He is happy and focused. Although no longer teammates or pursuing soccer careers, Scott and my son Keenan continue to be wonderful friends, supporting each other through their new journeys. Without a doubt, they will succeed.

JERRY

After less than a year in a wheelchair, Jerry began walking again with canes despite the lack of feeling in his legs, and he continues to work on being as mobile as his body is able. He and his first wife divorced but remain fast friends, and he is now in a fulfilling relationship. He is the very proud grandfather of five grandchildren—the lights of his life. He keeps busy managing a gift basket business for a local gourmet market and continues to be involved in dentistry, working as an expert witness in dental malpractice cases. He has never stopped traveling.

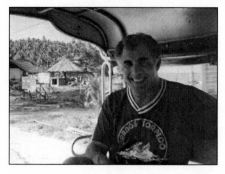

Jerry during his vacation

It has not been easy. Jerry lost a lot—his profession, his practice and participation in recreational activities he greatly enjoyed and daily routines he took for granted. Still, he does not harbor anger or any resentment.

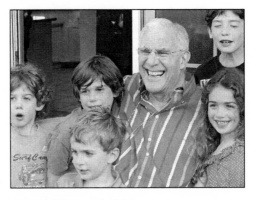

Jerry and his grandchildren

He moved on and made another full life for himself. He is loved and shares love. And service to others brings fulfillment to his life. He offers his advice and assistance to anyone who is in need. He will speak to them in person or over the phone about what to expect and how to deal with the unique issues associated with these types of physical problems. He will even visit their homes to help them organize the environment in order to function successfully, whatever it looks like. He will never stop. One of the most impressive and inspirational comments to come out of my research was made by Jerry. "I keep worrying I am not doing enough; I am not giving back enough," he said. That sums up the spirit of all of these survivors. Having the rug yanked out from under them, they adapted, moved on, focused on can instead of can't. And they gave back, continually.

DAVID

Once Allied soldiers liberated the Nazi concentrations camps, David was hospitalized. He had several medical problems due to his long, brutal interment. His sister Rachel, who escaped to England before the war, had met and married a pilot in the Royal Air Force. When the dust settled she sent him to search for her family. David was the only one he found.

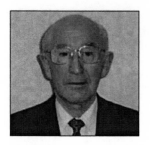

David

When David was done recuperating and moved to England, he experienced some anti-Semitism. But he carried on and went to school and became a pastry chef. He married, and he and his wife settled in London. He worked at several places but ended up at 10 Downing Street, where he had tea with Prime Minister Winston Churchill (who admired his pastries).

David eventually moved to the U.S. He and his wife had a son. David's wife passed away while they were living on the east coast, and he moved to the west coast, where he met and married his second wife, also a survivor. He spent time traveling around giving free public speeches about tolerance, sending a message to whoever would listen about love. Hatred, he said, causes so much tragedy, and we are really here to love and support each other.

In his later years, David was diagnosed with heart disease and needed surgery. One of the best cardiac surgeons available was of German descent. Knowing David's background, he had a respectful conversation with him. He disclosed his heritage and assured David that he was extremely competent and would take exceptionally good care of him. David agreed. He had moved forward and learned his own lesson: to love and trust no matter what.

I spoke with David on June 8, 2012. He is now 86 years old and has been giving talks for more than 26 years, the most recent just two weeks before we reconnected. He has slowed down, but he continues his mission: to promote tolerance and love. He and his wife thanked me for calling, and when I told them his story was in this book, he said, "I am so grateful." It never stops—always thoughtful gratitude. His stirring book, *Because of Romek*, is available for purchase at www.becauseofromek.com.

CONNIE

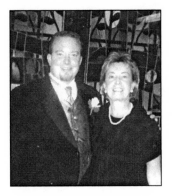

Connie and son, Matt, at his wedding

Connie has pitched for a softball team for 35 years, missing only one season—the one right after her accident. She is unbelievably active, recently playing four intense games in one weekend of a soccer tournament.

Probably her most amazing accomplishment since the accident was literally called "Climb Against the Odds." It was a hardcore hike up 14,179-foot Mt. Shasta—the fifth highest peak in California—to benefit the Breast Cancer Fund. She came within a few hundred feet of the top when foul weather struck and a boulder the size of a small car came crashing down. Her fellow climbers were sure the rock had killed her, but Connie emerged. Once again, she felt her guardian angel protected her.

When we caught up recently, she shared that 34 years ago that very day, she had her mastectomy. At the time, she thought she wouldn't live to see her children grow. That exact thought kept her alive after the crash in Croatia, and she has enjoyed many years of close, loving relationships with her son Matt and her daughter Stacey. She has traveled extensively to such places as Vietnam, Cambodia, Laos and Egypt. She celebrated Matt's wedding to his wife Toni on April 23, 2010. Most recently, she thrilled in Stacey's completion of a master's degree in humanities with honors and a special award for Outstanding Academic Achievement.

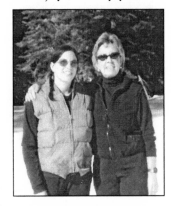

Connie and her daughter, Stacey

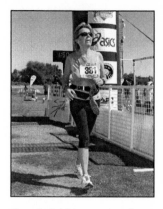

Connie finishing a race after her accident

To acknowledge that accomplishment, mother and daughter traveled to Thailand and Bali.

Connie never wants to forget those who helped and supported her in her recovery. And she is passionate about giving back. She focuses on homeless women and children, helping women at a shelter get back on their feet and gain employment. Her hospice work involves visiting people in need two to three times a week. She brings them a smile, reads out loud or just sits quietly next to them for comfort. She *needs* to be of service. She is getting all she can out of her own life by enriching the lives of those around her. She refuses to let the accident define her. It is how she lives her life now that defines her—a servant to others.

DOMINIC

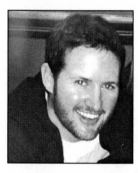

Dominic is an athlete. He has tremendous drive and a competitive spirit that has never waned. After graduating from the University of California, Berkeley he focused on his nonprofit organization Try For Others (tryforothers.org). He decided to widen the scope of what it could accomplish and the people it could serve. He reached out to all severely injured athletes, providing what equipment he could and sponsoring several in athletic events. In 2010, Try For Others began sponsoring the adaptive division of Eppie's Great Race, a run/bike/kayak team triathlon. Dominic noted the lack of incorporating adaptive athletes and spoke to the race's founder and director. He asked Dominic to be on the board, and in 2011, the race had its largest adaptive division since it began in 1974.

As he was building his nonprofit, Dominic rode a handcycle across the U.S. to bring attention to injured

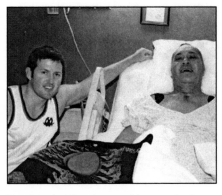

Dominic, helping through his organization

athletes and raise money for Try For Others. It became a passion. He has been racing, completing marathons and is an upcoming adaptive cyclist on the U.S. handcycling circuit. His ultimate goal in the sport is to compete in the 2016 Paralympics in Brazil.

Currently, he helps with the family business, which provides access solutions for the disabled and elderly. And he is following his passion for entrepreneurship by interning with the Sacramento Angels, an investment group that supports technology start-ups with seed funding and mentoring advice. His nonprofit continues to sponsor adaptive athletes, and he hopes to form a handcycling team in the future that would compete both nationally and internationally.

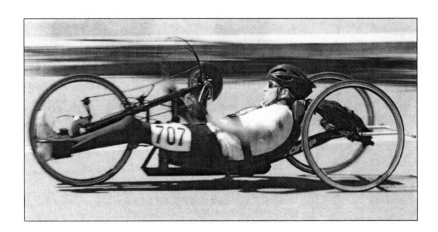

SUZY

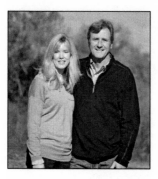

Suzy and her husband, Joe

For more than 15 years, Suzy has worked as the practice administrator for a very busy dermatological group. She is still in remission and an active force in her daughters' lives, having seen them through the completion of high school and college and into their busy lives in a variety of professions.

At this time, she is helping plan her eldest daughter's wedding. She and her husband Joe, who have been married for 28 years, have more time with each and enjoy traveling together on a regular basis. She has completed several Susan G. Komen Race for the Cure

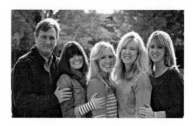

Suzy with her husband Joe and daughters, Amy, Molly, and Hillary

runs and can be seen running or walking with Joe on a regular basis. She loves life. It was rough, but she and her family, with love, support, optimism and incredible determination, overcame.

KURT

Although he has been affected by the current economic times, Kurt continually looks at the positive and lessons before him. There is a reason for everything; you just don't see it at the time, he says. After quitting a job he had for several years, he moved to Arizona to seek new employment and enjoy his favorite pastime, golf. He had a good life but missed his family, especially his son. To his surprise he was asked to resume his position as advertising manager for a California publication. He took the position and moved back home, to the delight of his family.

It has not always been smooth sailing, but through hard work and commitment Kurt has enjoyed successes personally and professionally. He is clear, however, that his proudest achievement is celebrating

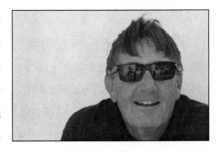

Kurt

24 years of being clean and sober, as of April 22, 2012. "I am a happy, active member of AA and continue on a path of sobriety," he says, adding that he continues to be "the father I always wanted" and diligently carries on his work with alcoholics hoping for better lives. "I am giving back what was so freely given to me."

FINALLY, ME

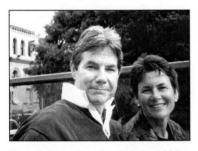

Terry & Joyce together in Italy, 1995

It has been many years since my accident, and many things, positive and not so positive, have happened. I have attended all of my children's major events, including graduations from high school and college. All were scholar athletes in Division 1 sports: Elizabeth played soccer at St. Mary's College and then for a semi-pro team. Catherine played water polo at Santa Clara University and then in Australia. Keenan played soccer at Marquette University and now is planning to go to film school.

I have seen both daughters get married to wonderful men, Elizabeth to Jake and Catherine to Patrick. I now have two grandchildren, with a third on the way. I love my role as grandmother, aka Mimi. Isabella and Brody are indeed lights of my life. They have been a salvation from some disturbing life issues more than

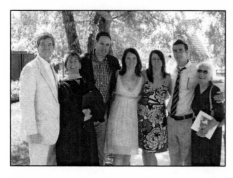

My graduation from St. Mary's—May, 2007

once, most recently the death of my dear mother, Mary Joyce Mikal. On November 29, 2010, she was found dead in her home. It was sudden and unexpected. She had been in good health. That same day my 35-year-old niece, Paula Marie, who had been fighting breast cancer died as well. Both of these events occurred on the Monday before Catherine's wedding. I went from planning my daughter's wedding to planning my mother's funeral, which took place a week later. And a week after that, Keenan graduated from Marquette, the same college my mother and father graduated from. My father Jude passed away nine years earlier, but we planned on having Grandma Mikal there to celebrate. It was not to be.

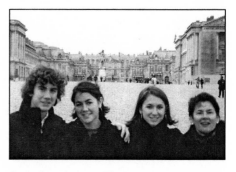

Catherine, Keenan, Elizabeth, and Joyce—Paris 2002

I had virtually no time to grieve or even process these events. Now both parents were gone and there was no will. I was assigned the task of administrating the estate and needed to organize six siblings immediately. It took a year to pull things together and bring forth a settlement for my brothers and sisters. Sometimes it was a bit contentious. During that time my husband decided to leave his job. I understood his decision, but it was unsettling. It was so much all at once. I was overwhelmed and lost. I talked to one of our favorite friends, Father Pat, who had given power-

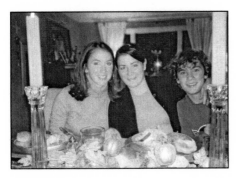

Elizabeth, Catherine, and Keenan— Thanksgiving, 2001

ful guidance in the past. I asked why God let this happen. I felt some of the same despair I had all those years ago. He reminded me that I was not without help. Sometimes God chooses to reveal Himself in different ways. Although we may feel that all is lost, all is taken, we are never without help. We do not need to struggle or go it alone. We are sent help and support—if we choose to recognize it.

I understood this intellectually, but I was still a bit lost. In January of 2012, I went out for my daily run. These runs are my time to think and pray. I was grieving the loss of my mother, worried about finances and wondering what happened to my life. I felt bitter and frustrated. All completely normal and understandable, I told myself. I deserved this resentment. As I continued to run and process, it occurred to me that there was a lot of energy in these negative thoughts and emotions. Then I thought, why don't I pour *that* energy into something productive? What about my book? I had put it aside to attend to other commitments and projects. Why not get moving on its completion and, instead of being angry, engage those I love in the process?

I got my husband involved. He is very bright and wonderful about getting things done. He took it all on and started moving things forward. My daughter Elizabeth worked in public

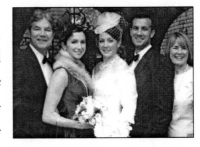

Catherine's Wedding—Dec. 3, 2010

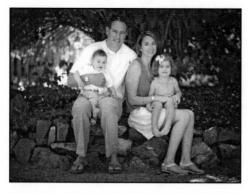

Elizabeth with husband, Jake, son, Brody, and daugher, Isabella

relations prior to having her children, and she was willing and able to help and came onboard. Keenan and Catherine listened to my ideas and read parts of the book, giving wonderful suggestions. It all came together, and as it did, my disillusion faded into urgency to get this book completed. I found absolute joy and peace working on it. As my friend reminded me, I was taking my own advice and turning tragedy into triumph.

Professionally, I have earned tenure and been promoted to associate professor at Sacramento State University. I have traveled to China, Wales and Ireland to discuss my research and published articles on the subject of MetaHabilitation. My husband is now happily employed. Elizabeth and Jake are expecting their third child. Catherine

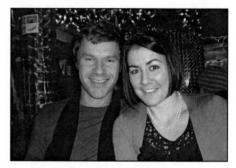

Catherine and husband, Patrick

and Patrick just moved to New York, as he graduated from medical school and is soon to begin his residency in emergency medicine. Keenan is moving to New York as well to work toward his goal in earnest. The book is done.

The stories in it are about lives that changed, sometimes drastically, and that continue to be challenging and imperfect. We can't always go back to the way things were. But change brings opportunities for other ways of being. We grieve the losses and eventually focus on the possibilities and move forward in big ways.

I am grateful. Having such a year was overwhelming, but once again, choosing to see things differently provided so many valuable lessons, opened up so many opportunities and reminded me to appreciate the life I have. It can be very scary and difficult, but as my daughter Catherine reminded me, "Mom, you never want to live your life coulda, woulda, shouda." I agree. I have been working on this idea for more than 15 years and this book for five. I am going for it. I hope you do, too.

REFLECTIONS

[We] may find meaning in life even when confronted by a ... fate that cannot be changed. For what matters then is to bare witness to the uniquely human potential at its best, which is to transform personal tragedy into a triumph. ... Suffering ceases to be suffering at the moment it finds a meaning.

—Viktor Frankl

This journey began for me on July 20, 1990. Having navigated through my own personal life crisis, studied and reflected on its meaning and challenges for many years, I have concluded that people can be exceptional. I saw what the event took from me, but more importantly, I weighed that against all that it gave me and revealed about who I had always been. I discovered this first in myself and later in others. I came across stories, patients, books, movies and plays that presented this same idea, that major life crisis is an opportunity, a fertile field for profound growth and development. And there is tremendous freedom in this opportunity.

One usually does not choose a personal life crisis. But his response is always a choice. That is the freedom. Thus the question becomes, if one is free to select more than one direction, why not choose MetaHabilitation? Survivors can regain a sense of hope and have faith that a significant future is possible despite their acute or long-term limitations. The decision is an enigma at times. I am not exactly certain, in all cases, why some move in this direction, but I am certain that they do. And when one bravely chooses the path of transforming a personal challenge into triumph and embraces the gifts provided by such an experience, he is enhanced in every possible way.

Nando Parrado said, "we all have our personal Andes." This was upon reflection, after he was far from the icy mountain where he and his rugby teammates endured horrifying conditions before somehow finding their way back to civilization and to life. He added: "I had been thinking of the disaster as a horrible mistake, as an unscripted deviation from the happy story of the life I had been promised." I felt this as well. Why me? I did everything right. It all seemed so unfair. However, as Nando acknowledged and I now understand, the "ordeal in the Andes was not an interruption of my true destiny, or a perversion of what my life was *supposed* to be. It simply *was* my life and the future that lay ahead was the only future that was available to me." Hiding from this reality or living in constant negativity, bitterness and anger prevents recognition of the gifts.

We go through a version of this process with lesser traumas or disruptions in our lives, but unfortunately, we do not always recognize them or pay attention to them as growth events. It is essential to learn from and recognize our strengths, even in the simplest of life's disruptions so that we are prepared, to some extent, to deal with the most profound existential angst brought on by ourselves or life itself. It is part of the gift one receives from these minor or major disruptions. Recognition and utilization of such events reminds us of our capacity and freedom to choose to grow in the face of adversity.

It is this assurance and absolute belief in humankind that I bring forward into my personal and professional life. The question at hand is how prepared are we, and what path do we take when confronted with these situations? How do we respond when life presents circumstances that we don't choose? The choice is to MetaHabilitate, to embrace the experience, to become engaged with what life has dealt you, to choose who you are and who you will be. Once you have chosen, then you must invest enormous effort and courage into seeing it through. It is essential to recognize that this choice is made within the limits the trauma has brought about. Many times we can't change outward conditions. But we can always decide how to react. We should always say yes within those confines.

My recovery was dependent on making this contribution to the field of rehabilitation. It has been a duty to create and promote the concept of MetaHabilitation. I have been changed by the experience of this investigation and work. It has allowed me to study an aspect of human behavior in depth, providing me with more understanding and appreciation of human potential and exactly what is brought forward by these unique existential experiences. Although some survivors and health care professionals take issue with the concept, I am enlightened and strengthened by what I have read and experienced, especially involving those I have interviewed, as well as countless friends and professional associates who have taken the time to discuss the infrastructure I'm trying to provide. These generative conversations and insights have brought about a conviction to promote this formative response to crisis, to push limits and eventually recognize the goodness brought forward by such events, understanding fully the reason for and necessity of a purposeful recovery.

I hold out great hope that the knowledge gained from this study will generate support for the concept and utilization of MetaHabilitation and stimulate further contemplation, discussion and work in this area. I see no acceptable alternative unless we are content with limiting human potential. I am not content. Steve Jobs agreed with this notion, declaring that death, and I would add crisis or trauma, is probably the best invention of life, calling it "life's change agent." His own life was short but incredible, and it touched billions of others. Any personal challenge has the potential to be such an invention or change agent, allowing one to face the danger but also recognize the opportunity.

I will never forget doing the research and interpreting the data into stages, characteristics and facilitating conditions. To be part of people's lives in such a special way—the interviews, the sharing of such intimate details—has had a profound impact on me personally and professionally. I feel blessed and honored to shed light on and give words to what these survivors accomplished so courageously.

Early on, during my high school years, I read Viktor Frankl's, *Man's Search for Meaning.* It was a class assignment. Sometime later, when visiting my favorite aunt – Aunt Betty, a very knowledgeable and wellread woman, I was reintroduced to this book. As Dominic told me, there are no coincidences. The seed was planted and has been growing for a very long time. I believe Frankl's writings have subconsciously driven my own thoughts and actions throughout my life. They have certainly made a difference during my journey of recovery and in this work.

It seems fitting to end with a provocative thought from Dr. Frankl:

As each situation in life represents a challenge to man and presents a problem for him to solve, the question of the meaning of life may actually be reversed. Thus, it is not man who asks the question, 'What is the meaning of life?' but he who is asked this question, for it is life itself that poses it to him. And man has to answer to life by answering for life; he has to respond by being responsible.

ACKNOWLEDGEMENTS

No one comes back from an event like mine without many, many wonderfully supportive and generous people. You picked me up, spiritually, mentally and emotionally when I could not go on. I am especially honored to acknowledge Drs. Bruce Gordon, Stuart Gherini, Garret Ryle and Mary Pat Petrich who brought me back to life. I am eternally grateful.

I would like to recognize Dr. Dan Fields, a friend and colleague who came to my rescue that day and has been instrumental in my journey back, personally and professionally. And Dr. Dan Van Hamersveld and the cardiac rehabilitation team at Sutter Hospital. You all gave me hope and supported my recovery showing me what I *could* do.

It is with great pleasure that I acknowledge and extend my sincere gratitude to Scott, Jerry, David, Dominic, Connie, Suzy, and Kurt. Sharing your unbelievably brave stories of metahabilitation helped create this new system and will assist others in times of trouble.

The decision to study and write about my experience and this new system of recovery took the time, effort and wonderful insights of many family, friends and colleagues who listened intently and helped process ideas and concepts. Thanks to all who took time to read the many versions of this manuscript, providing compelling comments and ideas of how to make this book just right.

I must acknowledge Dr. Dean Elias who took the time to read that first paper and reinforced the importance of this work. The hours spent refining the research and ideas are a gift I will always be tremendously grateful for. I am sure your remember I did not always agree or want to incorporate your suggestions, but each time I gave in and accepted those wise and thoughtful ideas -it just made it so much better.

I am especially grateful to Erin Ryan who wholeheartedly took on this venture and made it happen. You breathed life into this project when you told me: "not only can this book be written, it should be written." For all the revisions, refinements and reconsiderations – I extend my sincere appreciation.

Finally, I must acknowledge Dr. Bridget Parsh. A friend and colleague who consistently reminded me to finish this work, repeating time and time again, "is that a book done yet?" When I was about to give up, she took me aside and lovingly but sternly reminded me, "this is not about you. People *need* to hear what you have found out. They need this message."

Thanks Bridget.

DEFINITIONS

Healing

Healing has been defined as a complex, multidimensional process by which a person acquires the knowledge, skills and understanding to support current health and promote recovery. Additionally, the knowledge and enhanced understanding of the recovery process further facilitates recuperation by providing meaning of the lived experience (Frankl, 1992). Roy's Adaptation Model addresses physiological, psychological and spiritual adaptation prompting healing by recognizing changes in the environment, which stimulate the individual to make adaptive changes, prompting positive behavioral responses, including finding meaning in the event or illness. The knowledge serves to heighten an individual's health, quality of life and even dying with dignity (Roy & Andrews, 1991).

Rehabilitation

The current biomedical perspective views disease and illness as a malfunction of a biophysical mechanism with the limited goal of restoring one to a former capacity through rehabilitation; to bring a patient back to or close to baseline prior to the trauma, disease or surgical intervention. It seeks to simply return one to health, but that health is defined only as useful and constructive activity. This model does not address the intense psychosocial needs that result, nor does it frame the process as a vehicle for profound growth and intrapersonal understanding. Like so much of mainstream medicine, it is focused on the pathology and the physical facts rather than the emotions and possibilities.

MetaHabilitation

MetaHabilitation is an integrated understanding and approach, not only to the trauma from personal life crises and catastrophic events but more importantly, to the process of recovery. These events are opportunities that can initiate a multidimensional transformational process. It is a model and system built on the recognition of one's profound capacity to move beyond basic survival to find meaning and purpose in the trauma, which ultimately becomes a gift that provides the opportunity to creatively restructure yourself and your life.

Existentialism

Existentialism is grounded in man's existence and the *experience* of existence. Humans are motivated by a search for meaning in their existence—the human experience—including the immediacy, the perception and the meaning. Man is what he makes of himself, of his life, which is the first principle of existentialism according to Sartre (1967). It is not only the creation of meaning, but more importantly, recognition of the freedom to choose—to actively participate in the creation and search for meaning of their existence (Norcross, 1987). It allows and encourages mankind to give as much meaning to life and actualize as many human values as possible (Frankl, 1968).

Hardiness

Hardiness is a synonym of existential courage. It comprises firm, unyielding attitudes of commitment, control and challenge. It has been observed to augment performance and health in the presence of stressful changes, allowing one to improve perceptions and actions when deciding his future (Maddi, 2004).

SelfActualization

Selfactualization, according to Maslow (1970), is difficult to accurately explain: "It may loosely be described as the full use and exploitation of talents, capacities, potentialities and the like. Such people seem to be fulfilling themselves and to be doing the best that they are capable of doing, reminding us of Nietzsche's exhortation, 'Become what thou art!'" (p. 126). Maslow further describes selfactualized people as those "who have developed or are developing to the full stature of which they are capable." Self-actualization implies that gratification and/or conquest of the basic needs of safety, belongingness, love, respect and selfrespect and the cognitive needs for knowledge and understanding have occurred. "This is to say that all subjects felt safe and un-anxious, accepted, loved and loving, respectworthy and respected, and that they had worked out their philosophical, religious, or axiological bearings."

Transformation

Transformation is the act of changing in composition, structure or outward form or appearance—changing one configuration or expression into another. Transformation also refers to change in one's character, condition or nature, usually prompted by an internal or external force.

REFERENCES

Alligood, M. R., & Tomey, A. M. (2002). *Nursing theory, utilization and application.* St. Louis: Mosby-Year Book.

Faber, D. (2005). *Because of Romek: A holocaust survivor's memoir.* La Mesa, California: Faber Press. www.becauseofromek.com

Frankl, V. E. (1963). *Man's search for meaning: An introduction to logotherapy.* (I. Lasch, Trans.) New York: Washington Square Press.

Frankl, V. E. (1984). *Man's search for meaning; an introduction to logotherapy.* Boston: Beacon Press.

Frankl, V. E. (1992). *Man's search for meaning, an introduction to logotherapy.* Boston: Beacon Press.

Frankl, V. E. (1996). *Viktor Frankl – recollections: an autobiography.* (J. and J. Fabray, Trans). New York: Plenum Publishing.

Frankl, V. E. (2000). *Man's ultimate search for meaning.* Cambridge: Perseus.

Franz, C. (2002). St. Mary's College update. *St. Mary's College, 24,* 1-27.

Fredrick, M. (1998). *Fundamentals of anatomy and physiology.* New Jersey: Prentice Hall.

Frick, W. B. (1987). The symbolic growth experience: Paradigm for a humanistic-existential learning theory. *Journal of Humanistic Psychology, 27,* 406423.

Greening, T. (1964). Journal of Humanistic Psychology, www.tomgreening.com

Jobs, S. (2005). You've got to find what you love: Commencement address. *Stanford Report.* June 14.

Maddi, S.R. (2004). Hardiness: An operationalization of existential courage. *Journal of Humanistic Psychology, 44,* 279-298.

Maslow, A. (1987). *Motivation and personality.* New York: Harper & Row.

Maslow, A. (1976). *Religions, values, and peakexperiences.* New York: Penguin Group.

MikalFlynn, J. (1993). *A phenomenological study: Near death survivors.* Unpublished master's thesis, California State University, Sacramento, California.

Moustakas, C. (1977). *Turning points.* New Jersey: PrenticeHall, Inc.

Moustakas, C. (1990). *Heuristic research: design, methodology and applications.* Thousand Oaks: Sage Publications.

Newman, M.A. (1997). Evolution of Theory of Health as Expanding Consciousness. *Nursing Science Quarterly, 10,* 22-25.

Norcross, J. C. (1987). A rational and empirical analysis of existential psychotherapy. *Journal of Humanistic Psychology, 27,* 4168.

Parrado, N. (2006). *Miracle in the Andes.* Crown Publishers: New York.

Rogers, C. R. (1995). *On becoming a person.* Boston: Houghton Mifflin Company.

Roy, C., & Andrews, H. (1991). *The Roy adaptation model.* Connecticut: Appleton & Lange.

Sartre, J. (1967). *Existential psychoanalysis* (H. Barnes, Trans.). Chicago: Henry Regnery.

The MetaHab System

MetaHabilitation Manual

This short manual illustrates the model and mechanisms of MetaHabilitation. The six stages are reviewed and action plans suggested to help you move successfully through each stage and onto the next. It is essential to remember that after experiencing a trauma, being in a state of recovery is not an illness. It is not a psychological disorder. It is expected. Identifying it as such allows normalization of a healing process that often feels very abnormal.

MetaHabilitation's general concept involves cultivating thoughts and actions that prompt and inform basic recovery while allowing you to discover not only who you are but who you can be. It shows how to, over time, move past the struggle to appreciate the event for the insight it brings and the enhancements to attitudes and behaviors that happen as a result.

Moving forward in this trajectory allows no real turning back. As discussed earlier, you may slide back a bit, but there is never a return to the desperation you once felt. It is a way of thinking that allows you to take each personal life crisis, no matter how intense, and gradually bring forth a positive outcome. It is vital to note, as in my story and others, that getting through one crisis does not mean there are no more problems. Quite the contrary.

However, organizing and conducting our thoughts and actions in a productive, progressive manner fostered eventual acceptance and then mastery of our lives.

How do you take on each stage successfully in order to advance? Here are suggestions. Remember, each of you is an individual. Progress may look and feel different, but the goal is movement forward in your recovery.

Most importantly, do not be afraid to ask for help. Welcome it. It is not wise and certainly not productive or fun to go it alone. You need advice and outside perspective; just pick the right people to listen to. And as Dominic said, "trust your gut." When you amass enough information, make the call. Go for it! If you feel stuck, review the stage, facilitating conditions and characteristics and re-read the stories to give you inspiration.

Stage One

First things first. This is the time for all focus to be on immediate survival and acute care. With your energies consumed by the basics, family and other support systems must do what you cannot. In dire situations, when your very life may hang in the balance, they should find out about the critical care issues. Ask questions. Advocate. When speaking to MDs or RNs on your behalf, they should ask for information and guidance. Later, this will be turned over to you. For now, you may be trying to stay alive or recover acutely, so your family's job is to be your voice. They should generate questions and identify concerns in advance of meeting health care professionals. Everyone in the situation is a bit unnerved, so it's easy to forget things; writing them down in advance assists in communication and completeness of care. As does sharing information amongst the support group.

When your survival is assured, you can begin to look at the situation in terms of control. What are you able to control now? In the future? This list will change as you progress through the recovery process. It is critical to review and take charge of each area in which you have control; even little things make you feel less chaotic.

Next, make a list of things you perceive as beyond your control. Examine why. This provides perspective and enables reassessment of perceived lack of control. As time passes you will seek out more information, which brings opportunities for these aspects to change. You will always have more control than you are aware. Whether it is over thoughts, attitudes or specific treatments, recognize and wield it.

But this is not the time for your supporters to step away. Especially when survivors are out of the hospital and back at home or in a long-term rehabilitation facility, they begin to recognize deficiencies. This is a scary and confusing time, causing huge disruptions. Friends and family cannot be afraid to suggest and seek professional help. They and you can benefit from such professional help, starting with the grieving process. The life you all knew changed, sometimes drastically. Eventually a new life will open up. However, recognizing the change and all that comes with it causes panic and depression. There must be a letting go. Accept it as a stage, part of a process and not a permanent condition. Allowing grieving while working to find meaning allows productive activity and glimpses of a future.

Those overseeing your care should review with you and your advocates the facilitating conditions and characteristics of MetaHabilitation (see lists). If you have these, utilize them. If not identified in yourself or others, do not spend time criticizing perceived deficiencies; instead, recognize them as specific areas of intervention and behaviors to strive for as they guide you toward success. They are unambiguous clues and strategies used by survivors and families, profiled in this book, to move toward recovery and MetaHabilitation. It is not meant to be an exhaustive list. Feel free to add your own elements. More than likely there are unique strengths you used in the past, tools that allowed you to successfully navigate through troubling events and situations. Incorporate them again.

The following conditions are powerful supplements to the characteristics that promote MetaHabilitation:

- ☐ Family support, both initial and ongoing.
- ☐ Advocacy from family and support groups.
- ☐ Positive relationships with family and friends.
- ☐ Spirituality (a sense of a superior power from which to draw strength).
- ☐ Willingness, innate or learned, to accept help.
- ☐ Stay away from negative people and thoughts.
- ☐ Surround themselves with positive people and thoughts.
- ☐ Research conditions to receive the best and most up-to-date care.
- ☐ Go with their guts (make very personal decisions about their care and recovery).
- ☐ Exercise significant control over their care and recovery.
- ☐ Take time to grieve losses and figure things out.
- ☐ Accept their conditions—for now.
- ☐ Adapt to the situation and life.
- ☐ Recognize inner strength.
- ☐ Focus on what they still have and can still do, as well as the choices before them.
- ☐ Set goals, both short and long-term, allowing them to redesign their lives as they choose.
- ☐ Get back into life by taking one important step, and then another.
- ☐ Push limits (overcome fear and apprehension and try new things in an effort to improve).
- ☐ Contact others with similar problems to vent and give and receive encouragement.

☐ Give back (deep desire to make a difference).

☐ Maintain hope for the future.

☐ Recognize the gifts brought forth by the experience.

It is also important to note that there is some overlap between facilitating conditions and characteristics of the MetaHabilitated survivor. The latter includes the following:

☐ Grateful.

☐ Hopeful.

☐ Resilient.

☐ Optimistic.

☐ Surround themselves with positive, optimistic people.

☐ Adaptable.

☐ Refuse to live with anger and despair.

☐ Accepting.

☐ Grieve losses and life changes but ultimately move on.

☐ Stop asking, 'why me?' and instead ask, 'why not me?'

☐ Seek and accept help from others.

☐ Focus on possibilities (continally search for and are motivated by new opportunities).

☐ Keep their promises (use reassurances to others as motivation).

☐ Define themselves by their lives post-event rather than by the experience itself.

☐ Take time to contemplate past lives and build new ones.

☐ Insightful (able to gain wisdom about themselves and their conditions).

☐ Recognize and embrace personal choices.

☐ Review where they were, where they are now and where they want to go.

☐ Make sound and productive personal choices regarding care, goals and life.

☐ Give back.

Notes

_____

_____

_____

_____

_____

_____

_____

_____

_____

_____

_____

_____

_____

_____

_____

_____

_____

_____

_____

_____

_____

Stage Two

Once survival is assured you'll begin to make choices. Significant ones. The most significant is the choice to move forward. This is not easy or fearless. But it must be done if there is any chance for a meaningful life. Once made, all the work is directed in this manner--in the direction of success. As mentioned, survivors can almost remember the exact time and day when they said: "This is not fun; this is horrible, but I am choosing to move in this direction." They held onto hope and some of the slimmest optimism supported by those around them, and they said "yes" to life. It is not all better. There is a long way to go, but this is a defining moment. It changes everything. There are other decisions made as recovery happens, but this is the big one. I wrote mine down and remind myself of it on a regular basis. Why don't you do the same.

Notes

_____

_____

_____

_____

_____

_____

_____

_____

_____

_____

Stage Three

Now that you've said yes and are moving forward, take time with family and friends to look at any and all potential treatments. Be very optimistic but not foolish. Do not go with gimmicks that purport the quick fix. Be judicious in your efforts but try things--traditional and complementary medicine have much to offer. They are synergistic. One treatment modality is good, the other is as well, but together they can have an additive effect. Just make certain you communicate with all health care providers everything that you are doing to reduce the potential for adverse effects.

Enjoy successes. Don't focus on failures. Learn from them. BE OPTIMISTIC. And do what you can to keep the optimism building. It is not just a good idea; it works. Brain chemicals called neurotransmitters are affected, making you feel better and stronger. As Connie stated, "Thoughts become things. Think good ones. Choose good ones."

Do good things for yourself. Use whatever you have, spiritually, emotionally, mentally and physically to move forward. Become disciplined in your recovery efforts. Keep track of your time and review how far you have come and where you want to go. When you identify deficiencies, work on them. Don't criticize yourself. It is senseless and completely unproductive. Engage others in the effort. It gives you control, and when you continually focus on what you can do and how you are working to access or improve things you cannot, you feel less anxious and depressed. You are moving forward. List specific accomplishments, things you want to do in the future and precise plans to bring these to completion. As my colleague Dr. Bridget Parsh reminds me, the difference between people who succeed and those who do not is follow-through. If you list it, follow it through.

Notes

_____

_____

_____

_____

_____

_____

_____

_____

_____

_____

_____

_____

_____

_____

_____

_____

_____

_____

_____

_____

_____

Stage Four

Take a breath. Take some time to contemplate where you are and how far you have come. You have accepted and adapted--for now. It is time to reflect on all that has happened, a seeming whirlwind of emotional, physical and behavioral adjustments. You still have much to accomplish, but for now, stop. Get away. If you can, travel somewhere that you enjoy. Remove yourself from the familiar for awhile. Look around you. Are there places, even for short periods of time, that you can sit and think? Knowing that you must continue to work on yourself, accept what you have now and adapt. This is an internal job. So many people try to give advice, telling you what is good for you and what you need to do. They are trying to be helpful, but they cannot really know what you are feeling. Do some journaling. Just write things down. It doesn't have to make sense; it just needs to allow you to purge some pent up thoughts and feelings, including fears, hopes and surprises. All of the things you never thought you would get through or could get through and yet you did. Think about it. Write it down.

Notes

_____

_____

_____

_____

_____

_____

_____

_____

Stage Five

You have adapted, reflected, made adjustments and developed some understanding of what this crisis or trauma has meant; now it is time to move forward. At any level you can. Your life fell apart. The first three stages of MetaHabilitation allowed you to sit with the pieces and try to figure out where they all belonged. The fourth stage allowed you to look at each one and decide how to put them back together like Picasso did in his painting. Go with it. Take what you have and what you learned and move into a productive life. You may not look the same or act the same. You may have limitations to deal with, but choose, once again, to take on the challenges that lie ahead. You have a future. Rise above any real or perceived limitations and pour yourself into family, school, your job and society. Take time to write about what your life is like now. What are you grateful for? What do you see now that you did not understand before? What are you ready to take on? What did this crisis motivate you to do? You may be surprised. I know I was.

Notes

_____

_____

_____

_____

_____

_____

_____

_____

Stage Six

Now is the time to look at what you created--love the picture you put together. It makes perfect sense. You never wanted the crisis; you never signed up for trouble, but now you embrace its occurrence. You understand the lessons it brought, the relationships you appreciate so much more and opportunities taken instead of overlooked. You get it! Each day brings a new beginning. Lance Armstrong once said of his battle with cancer, "It is the best thing to happen to me, but I never want to go through that again." I have some issues with that notion of "best" but understand what he is pointing out. This trauma has given more gifts than it took away. I found a way to define my life, not as a result of it, but because of it. I focus on how I live my life after. I am in the now.

You have opportunities to contribute what you learned. The people in these stories took on such opportunities, finding them to be powerful parts of recovery--sometimes the most powerful. Giving back. It was contagious. Focus on your strengths. Be positive. Be thankful and cheerful and tell people you love them. Again, it is not just something nice to do; it changes who you are and those around you--in a big way. Try it.

I see life so differently now. As Dominic and I discussed, sometimes it's hard to hold onto the lessons. Life, once again, gets in the way, but I refuse to let it take over. I don't ask what life is about. I tell life, as Frankl suggested, this is what you are about. Take on your future. I have a mission. This book is one of them. What is yours?

Notes

About the Author

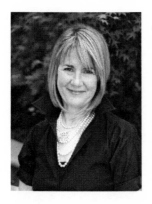 Joyce Mikal-Flynn survived after 22 minutes of CPR. She is an avid runner, a mother of three and a grandmother has completed several marathons and triathlons before and after she suffered a sudden cardiac arrest. She holds a Bachelor of Science in Nursing from the University of San Francisco and a Nurse Practitioner credential from the University of California, Davis. She earned a Master of Science in Nursing from Sacramento State University and a Doctor of Education from St. Mary's College of California *after* her accident. She continues her Nurse Practitioner practice and is an Associate Professor at Sacramento State University in the School of Nursing. A sought after motivational speaker, she continues to write and present her research on MetaHabilitation nationally and internationally.

Contact her at: jmikalflynn@comcast.net or MetaHab.com.